AF179651

DORLAND'S CARDIOLOGY SPELLER

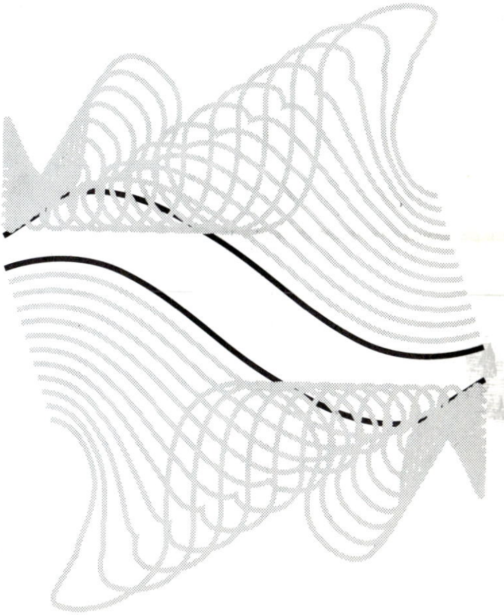

Consultants

DAVID J. SKORTON, MD
Professor and Associate Chair for Clinical Programs,
Department of Internal Medicine,
College of Medicine;
Professor, Department of Electrical and
Computer Engineering,
College of Engineering,
The University of Iowa

MICHAEL KIENZLE, MD
Associate Professor of Medicine and
Assistant Director, Cardiovascular Division,
Department of Internal Medicine,
The University of Iowa College of Medicine,
Iowa City, Iowa

Consultant for Syllabication

CAROL A. HART, PhD
Narberth, Pennsylvania

DORLAND'S CARDIOLOGY SPELLER

W.B. SAUNDERS COMPANY
Harcourt Brace Jovanovich, Inc.
Philadelphia London Toronto Montreal Sydney Tokyo

W. B. SAUNDERS COMPANY
Harcourt Brace Jovanovich, Inc.

The Curtis Center
Independence Square West
Philadelphia, Pennsylvania 19106

Library of Congress Cataloging-in-Publication Data

Dorland's cardiology speller.

p. cm.

ISBN 0–7216–3748–5

1. Cardiology—Terminology. I. W.B. Saunders Company. II. Title: Cardiology speller. [DNLM: 1. Cardiology—nomenclature. WG 15 D711]

RC666.3.D67 1992 616.1′2′0014—dc20

DNLM/DLC 92–13385

Dorland's Cardiology Speller ISBN 0–7216–3748–5

Copyright © 1992 by W. B. Saunders Company

All rights reserved. No part of this publication may be reproduced or transmitted in any form or by any means, electronic or mechanical, including photocopy, recording, or any information storage and retrieval system, without permission in writing from the publisher.

Printed in United States of America.

Last digit is the print number: 9 8 7 6 5 4 3 2 1

Preface

As the foundation of medical knowledge increases in depth and breadth, the rate of acquisition of knowledge increases ever more rapidly, and consequently the vocabulary of medicine is constantly expanding and changing. Even within individual specialties, the body of terminology is both voluminous and subject to continual modification. No dictionary can include all of the many disorders, procedures, types of apparatus, techniques, therapies, tests, and pharmaceuticals, or all of the terms describing physiology, histology, and anatomy relevant to a particular specialty. Hence, *Dorland's Cardiology Speller* has been created to provide in a single reference relevant entries from the *Dorland's Illustrated Medical Dictionary* database as well as terms culled from textbooks, reference books, and medical journals. As a word list, it can contain many entries too restricted in scope for inclusion in a general dictionary, while excluding words unlikely to be encountered regularly in the field of cardiology.

Terms are arranged as a single alphabetic list, with eponymic terms also listed under each of the proper names and hard to find terms given multiple listings. As many pharmaceutical trademarks and eponymic entries have been included as possible, since these words are the ones most likely to have idiosyncratic spellings. Other frequently encountered trademarks have also been included; most describe cardiac valves, pacemakers, and electrocardiography equipment. In addition, acceptable end of line syllable breaks are provided, a feature that can be very difficult to find for specialized medical words.

Our thanks go to our consultants, David J. Skorton, MD, and Michael Kienzle, MD, who reviewed the word list, and to our consultant for syllabication, Carol A. Hart, PhD, for their valuable work.

PATRICIA D. NOVAK, PHD
Lexicographer

How This Book Is Arranged

Order of Entries

Dorland's Cardiology Speller follows the same scheme of arrangement as *Dorland's Illustrated Medical Dictionary*. Main entries follow one another in letter-by-letter alphabetical order regardless of spaces or hyphens that occur within them (see below for special rules for chemical names); compound entries consisting of one or more adjectives and a noun will be found as subentries under the noun.

In some cases where there might be a question about where to look to find an entry, entries have been given in more than one place, even under an adjective.

Eponymic terms. Terms containing a proper name are give multiple listings, once under the thing named and once under each eponym. Thus *Adams-Stokes syncope* is listed as:

syncope
  Adams-Stokes s.

Adams
  A.-Stokes syncope

Stokes
  Adams-S. syncope

Terms containing a proper name that occurs in several forms, such as *von Willebrand/Willebrand,* will be listed under each alternative form:

von Willebrand
  v.W. syndrome

Willebrand
  W. syndrome

Umlauts are ignored for alphabetization, and proper names beginning *Mc* or *Mac* are alphabetized as though spelled *Mac.*

Chemical prefixes. Italicized chemical prefixes such as the letters *p*- and *o*- and *cis*- and *trans*-, together with numbers, Greek letters, and the small capitals L- and D-, do not count for alphabetization. When prefixes are written out in full, however, as *para-* instead of *p-*, they are counted for alphabetical order.

Subentries

Each subentry appears on a new line following the main entry and is indented. The main entry word in a subentry is represented only by the initial letter as *mast c.* (under *cell*), with three exceptions. For regular English plurals, the abbreviation is the initial letter followed by *'s* (as *m's* for *muscles*). For irregular or Greek or Latin plurals, the entire plural form is written out (as *indices* under *index* and *venae* under *vena*). For possessive forms, the initial letter is followed by *'s* (as *A's disease* for *Albright's disease*). In subentries the main entry word is ignored for alphabetization, as are prepositions, conjunctions, and articles.

Possessive Forms

The use of the possessive in eponyms is controversial. This book follows the example of *Dorland's Illustrated Medical Dictionary,* that is, the *'s* is favored where the sources for a term justify its appearance. Whether or not to use the possessive form is a matter left to the individual; owing to the present lack of consistency and consensus, no prescription can be given. There are of course some terms in which the possessive is never used, as *Down syndrome.*

Abbreviations and Acronyms

A number of abbreviations and acronyms are given, together with the words or phrases that they stand for. The selection is of course only a small fraction of the abbreviations and acronyms in actual use. If more than one word or phrase is listed with an abbreviation, the terms are given in alphabetical order and each additional term is placed on a new line and indented.

Word Divisions

Acceptable word divisions are given for main entries; syllabication is based on pronunciation. Not all syllable breaks are shown; for example, because single letters at the beginnings and ends of words may not be separated from the rest of the word, such divisions are not given. Likewise, single letters should not be separated from the word elements they belong to in compound words. Breaks that could confuse the reader as to the meaning of a word are to be avoided. In many cases, words may be broken at other places than the ones that appear in this book (for example, different pronunciations imply different word breaks); it is impossible to show every break that could occur for every word. What appears here is one possible system.

Alternative Spellings

A number of words have alternative spellings, ranging from the difference of a single letter to the use of variant forms of Greek and Latin stems. Although every effort has been made to ensure that the spellings included in this book are valid, no indications of preference are given.

Brackets and Parentheses

Some entries require a bit of explanation; these explanations are enclosed in parentheses. Brackets are sometimes used as a part of Latin anatomical nomenclature to enclose an eponym in the genitive case; in this book such eponyms generally appear all lower case (as in *Dorland's Illustrated Medical Dictionary*) but an initial capital for the name is acceptable.

Plurals

Plurals for foreign words, nearly all of them Greek and Latin, are given with the appropriate entries. In addition, they are given again as separate entries if they do not occur within a few lines of the singular form.

A

A
  ampere
  atrium

A
  area

A_1
  aortic first heart sound

A_2
  aortic second sound

AII
  angiotensin II

a.
  L. arteria (artery)

AA
  ascending aorta

aa.
  L. arteriae (arteries)

AAA
  abdominal aortic aneurysm
  abdominal aortic aneurysmectomy

α_2PI
  alpha$_2$-antiplasmin

AAI (atrial demand inhibited) pace•maker

AAI (atrial inhibited) pac•ing

AA in•ter•val

AAIR (atrial demand inhibited–rate responsive) pace•maker

AAI-RR (atrial demand inhibited–rate responsive) pace•maker

Aase syndrome

AAT (atrial demand triggered) pace•maker

AAT (atrial triggered) pac•ing

A band

ABC
  airway, breathing, and circulation

ab•er•ran•cy
  acceleration-dependent a.
  bradycardia-dependent a.
  deceleration-dependent a.
  phase 3 a.
  phase 4 a.
  tachycardia-dependent a.

ab•er•ra•tion
  intraventricular a.
  postextrasystolic a.

abeta•lipo•pro•tein•emia

Abi•plat•in

Abi•trate

ab•la•tion
  electrical a.
  radio frequency a.

ab•nor•mal•i•ty
  juvenile ST segment a.
  left atrial a.

abouche•ment

ab•scess
  brain a.
  myocardial a.

acan•tho•cy•to•sis

ACAT
  acyl CoA:cholesterol acyltransferase
  automatic computerized axial tomography

ACC
  American College of Cardiology

ac•cen•tu•a•tion
presystolic a.

ac•cre•tio
a. cordis
a. pericardii

Ac•cur•bron

ACE
angiotensin-converting enzyme

ac•e•bu•to•lol

acet•a•min•o•phen

Ace•taz•o•lam

ac•et•a•zol•a•mide
a. sodium

ac•e•tyl•cho•line

N-ac•e•tyl•pro•cain•amide

ac•e•tyl•sal•i•cyl•ic acid

ac•e•tyl•stro•phan•thi•din

ac•id
acetylsalicylic a.
adenylic a.
aminocaproic a.
p-aminosalicylic a.
arachic a.
arachidic a.
arachidonic a.
ascorbic a.
bile a's
butanoic a.
butyric a.
capric a.
caproic a.
caprylic a.
chenodeoxycholic a.
cholaic a.
cholanic a.
choleic a's
cholic a.
citric a.
clupandonic a.
crotonic a.
dehydrocholic a.

ac•id *(continued)*
deoxycholic a.
diethylenetri-aminepentaacetic a.
digammacarboxy-glutamic a.
docosahexaenoic a.
eicosanoic a.
eicosapentaenoic a.
erucic a.
essential fatty a's
ethacrynic a.
ethylenediamine-tetraacetic a.
fatty a.
n-3 fatty a's
ω-3 fatty a's
ω-6 fatty a's
folic a.
fusidic a.
gammacarboxyglutamic a.
glycochenodeoxycholic a.
glycocholic a.
heptadecanoic a.
hexadecanoic a.
hexanoic a.
hydrocyanic a.
hydroperoxyeicosatet-raenoic a.
hydroxyeicosatetraenoic a.
hydroxyheptadeca-trienoic a.
icosanoic a.
lactic a.
lauric a.
linoleic a.
linolic a.
lithocholic a.
mevalonic a.
monounsaturated fatty a's
myocardial fatty a.
myristic a.
nicotinic a.
nonesterified fatty a's
octadecanoic a.
octanoic a.
oleic a.
omega-3 fatty a's

ac•id *(continued)*
omega-6 fatty a's
palmitic a.
palmitoleic a.
para-aminosalicylic a.
phosphatidic a.
polyglycolic a.
polyunsaturated fatty a's
pyruvic a.
ricinoleic a.
saturated fatty a.
stearic a.
taurochenodeoxycholic a.
taurocholic a.
tetracosanoic a.
unsaturated fatty a.
uric a.
ursodeoxycholic a.
vaccenic a.

ac•i•de•mia

ac•i•do•sis
metabolic a.

ac•i•dot•ic

ac•id•uria
orotic a.

Aci•ne•to•bac•ter
A. calcoaceticus

acleis•to•car•dia

ac•quired im•mu•no•de•fi•cien•cy syn•drome (AIDS)

ac•qui•si•tion
gated a.

ac•ro•ceph•a•lo•syn•dac•ty•ly

ac•ro•meg•a•ly

acrot•ic

ac•ro•tism

ACS
American Cancer Society
American College of Surgeons

ACT
activated clotting time

ACTH
adrenocorticotropic hormone

Ac•thar

ac•tin

Ac•tino•ba•cil•lus
A. actinomycetemcomitans

Ac•ti•no•my•ces
A. israelii

ac•ti•no•my•co•sis

ac•tion
ball-valve a.
capillary a.

ac•ti•va•tion
blood cell a.
chamber a.
complement a.
length-dependent a.
ventricular a.
ventriculoatrial a.

ac•ti•va•tor
fibrin-specific plasminogen a.
recombinant tissue plasminogen a.
single chain urokinase-type plasminogen a.
tissue plasminogen a. (t-PA, TPA)
tissue-type plasminogen a.

ac•tiv•i•ty
electrical a.
intrinsic sympathomimetic a.
malignant ventricular ectopic a.
physical a.
plasma post-heparin lipolytic a.
sustained rhythmic a.
triggered a.

acy•clo•vir

ac•yl cho•les•ter•ol ac•yl•trans•fer•ase

ac•yl CoA
  acyl coenzyme A

ac•yl CoA:cho•les•ter•ol ac•yl•trans•fer•ase

ac•yl co•en•zyme A

ac•yl•glyc•er•ol

ac•yl-SK
  acyl-streptokinase

N-ac•yl•sphin•go•sine

acyl-strep•to•ki•nase

Ad•a•lat

Adam•kie•wicz
  arteries of A.

Ad•ams
  A. disease
  A.-DeWeese device
  A.-Stokes attack
  A.-Stokes disease
  A.-Stokes syncope
  A.-Stokes syndrome
  Morgagni-A.-Stokes syndrome
  Stokes-A. attack
  Stokes-A. syncope
  Stokes-A. syndrome

Ad•ap•in

adap•ter
  catheter a.
  lead a.
  syringe a.

ADC
  analog-to-digital converter

Ad•di•son
  A's disease

Adeno•card

ad•e•no•ma
  adrenal a.

aden•o•sine
  a. monophosphate (AMP)
  a. triphosphate (ATP)

aden•o•sine de•am•i•nase

aden•o•sine•tri•phos•pha•tase

ad•e•no•vi•rus

aden•yl•ate cy•clase

ad•e•nyl•ic acid

ADH
  antidiuretic hormone

adi•emor•rhy•sis

ad•i•po•cyte

ad•i•po•gen•e•sis

ad•i•po•gen•ic

ad•i•pog•e•nous

ad•i•poid

ad•i•po•kin•e•sis

ad•i•po•kin•et•ic

ad•i•pol•y•sis

ad•i•po•lyt•ic

ad•i•pom•e•ter

ad•i•po•pex•is

ad•i•pose

ad•i•po•sis
  a. universalis

ad•i•pos•i•tas
  a. cordis

ad•re•nal

Adren•a•lin

ad•re•ner•gic
  α-a.
  alpha-a.

ad•re•ner•gic *(continued)*
  β-a.
  beta-a.

adre•no•cep•tor
  alpha a.
  beta a.

adre•no•cor•ti•coid

adre•no•gen•i•tal syn•drome

Adri•a•my•cin

Adru•cil

Ad•son
  A. forceps

ad•ster•nal

Ad•vantz DX digital system

AEC (ankyloblepharon-ectodermal dysplasia-clefting) syn•drome

aer•emia

Aero•coc•cus

aero•em•bo•lism

Aero•late

Aero•lone

aer•o•sol
  radiolabeled a.

AF
  atrial fibrillation
  atrial flutter

af•fer•en•tia

AFib
  atrial fibrillation

A fib
  atrial fibrillation

AFL
  atrial flutter

AFl
  atrial flutter

af•ter•de•po•lar•iza•tion
  delayed a.
  early a.
  late a.

af•ter•load
  a. matching
  a. mismatching
  ventricular a.

af•ter•po•ten•tial

Ag
  silver (L. argentum)

agent
  α-adrenergic blocking a.
  β-adrenergic blocking a.
  adrenergic blocking a.
  adrenoceptor blocking a.
  alpha-adrenergic blocking a.
  antianginal a.
  antiarrhythmic a.
  antidiabetic a.
  antihypertensive a.
  antiinflammatory a.
  antiplatelet a.
  antipsychotic a.
  antituberculous a.
  beta-adrenergic blocking a.
  beta-blocking a.
  calcium channel–blocking a.
  cardiotropic a.
  cerebroprotective a.
  chemotherapeutic a.
  contrast a.
  hemostatic a.
  inhalation a.
  inotropic a.
  microbubble contrast a.
  nonglycoside inotropic a.
  nonsteroidal antiinflammatory a.
  pressor a.
  sympathomimetic a.
  topical hemostatic a.
  unloading a.

agent *(continued)*
vagomimetic d.
vasoactive a.
viral a.

ag•ger *pl.* ag•ge•res
a. valvae venae

ag•gre•ga•tion
platelet a.

agly•con

AGN
acute glomerulonephritis

ag•o•nist
adrenergic a.
α-adrenergic a.
$beta_2$-a.

agran•u•lo•cy•to•sis

am•i•ka•cin
a. sulfate

Ah
ampere-hour

AHA
American Heart Association

A–H in•ter•val

A-hydro•Cort

AICD
automatic implantable cardioverter-defibrillator

AIDS
acquired immunodeficiency syndrome

air en•trap•ment syn•drome

air•way
esophageal obturator a.
oropharyngeal a.

AIVR
accelerated idioventricular rhythm

ak•i•ne•sia

ak•i•ne•sis

ak•i•net•ic

Ak-Zol

Al
aluminum

ALAD
abnormal left axis deviation

Ala•gille
A's syndrome

al•a•nine

al•a•nine ami•no•trans•fer•ase

Al•bi•ni
A's nodules

Al•bright
A's disease
A's syndrome
A.-McCune-Sternberg syndrome
McCune-A. syndrome

al•bu•min
technetium Tc 99m aggregated a.

al•bu•min•uria

al•bu•ter•ol
a. sulfate

al•co•hol
ethyl a.
steroid a.

Al•dac•tone

Al•do•met

al•do•ster•one

al•do•ster•on•ism

Al•ex•an•der
A. rib raspatory
A. rib stripper

al•fen•ta•nil

ALG
  antilymphocyte globulin

al•gio•vas•cu•lar

al•go•vas•cu•lar

ali•as•ing

alipo•gen•ic

ali•poi•dic

alipo•trop•ic

Al•ka-Bu•ta•zol•i•din

Al•ka•bu•ta•zone

al•ka•line phos•pha•tase

al•ka•lo•sis
  metabolic a.

Al•ka-Phen•yl•bu•ta•zone

al•kap•ton•uria

Al•len
  A's test
  A. key
  Bloor, Pelkan, and A's method

Al•lis
  A. clamp

Al•li•son
  A. lung retractor

al•lo•ge•ne•ic

al•lo•gen•ic

al•lo•graft
  cardiac a.

al•lo•rhyth•mia

al•lo•rhyth•mic

all or none

al•lo•trans•plan•ta•tion

al•loy
  Elgiloy a.

ALP
  alkaline phosphatase

al•pha-ac•ti•nin

al•pha-ad•re•ner•gic

al•pha-a•go•nist

al•pha-lipo•pro•tein

al•pha-meth•yl•do•pa

al•pha$_2$ PI
  alpha$_2$-plasmin inhibitor

al•pha$_2$-plas•min in•hib•i•tor

al•pha-stat

Al•port
  A's syndrome

al•pra•zo•lam

al•pren•o•lol
  a. hydrochloride

ALT
  alanine aminotransferase

AL•ter•na•GEL

al•ter•nans
  cardiac a.
  electrical a.
  a. of the heart
  mechanical a.
  pulsus a.
  QRS a.
  ST segment a.
  T wave a.
  total a.
  total electrical a.
  U wave a.

al•ter•na•tion
  cardiac a.
  electrical a. of the heart

Alu-Cap

alu•mi•num
  a. hydroxide
  a. oxide

Alu-Tab

Al•za•pam

Amer•i•can Can•cer So•ci•e•ty

Amer•i•can Col•lege of Car•di•ol•o•gy

Amer•i•can Col•lege of Nu•cle•ar Phy•si•cians

Amer•i•can Col•lege of Sur•geons

Amer•i•can Heart As•so•ci•a•tion

Amer•i•can So•ci•e•ty of Hy•per•ten•sion

Amer•sol

Am•i•car

am•i•do•tri•zo•ate
sodium a.

Am•i•kin

amil•o•ride
a. hydrochloride

amine
sympathomimetic a.

ϵ-ami•no•ca•pro•ic acid

ami•no•gly•co•side

Ami•noph•yl•lin

am•i•noph•yl•line

6-ami•no-D-psi•co•fu•ra•no•syl•pu•rine

amin•o•rex
a. fumarate

p-ami•no•sal•i•cyl•ic acid

ami•o•da•rone

Am•i•paque

am•i•trip•ty•line
a. hydrochloride

am•mo•nia
a. N (nitrogen) 13

am•mo•ni•um
a. chloride

amox•a•pine

amox•i•cil•lin

Amox•il

AMP
adenosine monophosphate

am•pere-hour

am•phi•cen•tric

Am•pho•jel

am•pho•ter•i•cin B

amp•i•cil•lin

Am•platz
A. coronary catheter
A. technique

am•pli•fi•er
atrial a.
ventricular sensing a.

am•pli•tude
pulse a.

am•ri•none

am•sa•crine

Amsa P-D

Am•si•dyl

am•y•loi•do•sis
cardiac a.
familial a.
senile a.

ANA
antinuclear antibodies

an•a•crot•ic

anac•ro•tism

an•al•ge•sia
bilateral intrapleural regional a.

an•al•ge•sic
narcotic a.

an•a•logue
glucose a.

an•al•pha•lipo•pro•tein•emia

anal•y•sis *pl.* anal•y•ses
bayesian a.
blood gas a.
computerized image a.
pacing system a.
Sonoclot a.
vector a.
videodensitometric a.
wall motion a.

an•a•ly•zer
blood gas a.
oxygen gas a.
pacing system a.
pulse height a.
Vitatron impulse a.

ana•phy•la•tox•in

ana•phy•lax•is

anas•to•mose

an•as•to•mo•sis *pl.* an•as•to•mo•ses
arteriovenous a.
Blalock-Taussig a.
heterocladic a.
homocladic a.
portacaval a.
portosystemic a.
systemic-pulmonary a.
terminoterminal a.

Ana•var

An•ca•lix•ir

An•cef

An•co•bon

An•co•til

an•crod

An•der•son
A.-Fabry disease

An•drews
A. suction tip

an•dro•gen

AN-DTPA

An•ec•tine

ane•mia
acute a.
aplastic a.
chronic hemolytic a.
congenital hypoplastic a.
Cooley's a.
Fanconi's a.
hemolytic a.
hemolytic a., microangiopathic
Mediterranean a.
megaloblastic a.
sickle cell a.
a. splenetica
splenic a.

An•er•gan

An•es•ta•con

An•es•ta•tal

an•es•the•sia
epidural a.
general a.
lytic cocktail a.
regional a.

an•es•the•si•ol•o•gist

an•es•thet•ic
general a.
regional a.

an•eu•rysm
abdominal a.
abdominal aortic a.
ampullary a.
aortic a.
aortic sinusal a.
arteriovenous a.

an•eu•rysm *(continued)*
arteriovenous pulmonary a.
ascending aortic a.
atherosclerotic a.
bacterial a.
berry a.
brain a.
cardiac a.
cerebral a.
cirsoid a.
compound a.
cylindroid a.
dissecting a.
dissecting aortic a.
ectatic a.
embolic a.
false a.
fusiform a.
hernial a.
infected a.
innominate a.
intracranial a.
lateral a.
miliary a.
mycotic a.
mycotic aortic a.
orbital a.
Park's a.
pelvic a.
Pott's a.
racemose a.
Rasmussen's a.
renal a.
Richet's a.
Rodrigues' a.
ruptured a.
saccular a.
sacculated a.
serpentine a.
suprasellar a.
syphilitic a.
syphilitic aortic a.
thoracic a.
traumatic a.
true a.
tubular a.
varicose a.

an•eu•rysm *(continued)*
venous a.
ventricular a.

an•eu•rys•mal

an•eu•rys•mat•ic

an•eu•rys•mec•to•my

an•eu•rys•mo•plas•ty

an•eu•rys•mor•rha•phy

an•eu•rys•mot•o•my

ANF
atrial natriuretic factor

An•ger
A. camera
A. gamma camera

an•gi•al•gia

an•gi•as•the•nia

an•gi•ec•ta•sis

an•gi•ec•ta•tic

an•gi•ec•to•my

an•gi•ec•to•pia

ang•i•itis *pl.* an•gi•it•i•des
leukocytoclastic a.
necrotizing a.
visceral a.

an•gi•na
a. cordis
crescendo a.
a. cruris
a. decubitus
exertional a.
a. inversa
nonexertional a.
a. pectoris
a. pectoris electrica
a. pectoris vasomotoria
preinfarction a.
Prinzmetal's a.
progressive a. pectoris
a. sine dolore
stable a.

an•gi•na *(continued)*
stable a. pectoris
unstable a.
variant a.
variant a. pectoris
vasomotor a.

an•gi•nal

an•gin•i•form

an•gi•noid

an•gi•nose

an•gi•no•sis

an•gi•nous

an•gio•ac•cess

an•gio•as•the•nia

an•gio•atax•ia

an•gio•car•dio•gram

an•gio•car•di•og•ra•phy
equilibrium a.
equilibrium radionuclide a.
exercise radionuclide a.
first pass a.
first pass radionuclide a.
gated equilibrium radionuclide a.
radionuclide a.

an•gio•car•dio•ki•net•ic

an•gio•car•di•op•a•thy

an•gio•car•di•tis

An•gio•cath catheter

An•gio-Con•ray

an•gi•odyn•ia

an•gio•ec•tat•ic

an•gio•gen•ic

an•gio•gram

an•gio•graph

an•gi•og•ra•phy
cine a.
coronary a.
digital subtraction a.
exercise radionuclide a.
intra-arterial digital subtraction a.
intravenous digital subtraction a.
pulmonary a.
pulmonary wedge a.
radionuclide a.

an•gio•he•mo•phil•ia

an•gio•hy•a•li•no•sis

an•gio•in•va•sive

an•gio•ker•a•to•ma
a. corporis diffusum

an•gio•ki•ne•sis

an•gio•ki•net•ic

an•gio•li•po•ma

an•gio•lo•gia

an•gi•ol•o•gy

an•gi•o•ma
cardiac a.

an•gio•ne•cro•sis

an•gio•neu•rec•to•my

an•gio•neu•ro•path•ic

an•gio•neu•rop•a•thy

an•gio•neu•rot•o•my

an•gio•no•ma

an•gio•pa•ral•y•sis

an•gio•pa•re•sis

an•gi•op•a•thy

an•gio•plas•ty
balloon a.
coronary a.
excimer laser a.
laser a.

an•gio•plas•ty *(continued)*
laser thermal a.
percutaneous transluminal a.
percutaneous transluminal coronary a.
transluminal coronary a.

an•gi•or•rha•phy
arteriovenous a.

an•gio•sar•co•ma
cardiac a.

an•gio•scle•ro•sis

an•gio•scle•rot•ic

an•gi•os•co•py
fiberoptic a.

an•gio•spasm

an•gio•spas•tic

an•gio•ste•no•sis

an•gi•os•te•o•sis

an•gi•o•sthe•nia

an•gi•os•to•my

an•gio•te•lec•ta•sis *pl.* an•gio•te•lec•ta•ses

an•gio•ten•sin
a. II

an•gio•ten•sin-con•vert•ing en•zyme

an•gi•ot•o•my

an•gio•to•nia

an•gio•ton•ic

an•gio•troph•ic

An•gio•vist

an•gle
cardiodiaphragmatic a.
cardiophrenic a.
phrenopericardial a.
Pirogoff's a.
sternal a.

an•gle *(continued)*
a. of sternum
venous a.

an•gor
a. pectoris

an•gu•lus *pl.* an•gu•li
a. Ludovici
a. sternalis
a. sterni
a. venosus

An•hy•dron

Anich•kov
A's cell
A's myocyte

an•ion
superoxide a.

an•is•in•di•one

an•iso•pi•esis

an•iso•trop•ic

AN-MAA

an•nu•lo•aor•tic

an•nu•lo•plas•ty
DeVega a.
mitral a.

an•nu•lor•rha•phy

an•nu•lus *pl.* an•nu•li
aortic a.
aortic valve a.
atrioventricular annuli
atrioventricular valve annuli
annuli fibrosi cordis
mitral a.
mitral valve a.
a. ovalis
pulmonary a.
pulmonary valve a.
tricuspid a.
tricuspid valve a.
valve a.
Vieussens' a.

an•ode

anom•a•ly
  cardiac a's
  Ebstein's a.
  Uhl's a.

an•orex•ia
  a. nervosa

anox•ia
  myocardial a.

ANP
  atrial natriuretic peptide

AN re•gion

An•rep effect

An•spor

AN-Sul•fur Col•loid

ANT
  anterior

ant•ac•id

an•tag•o•nism
  accentuated a.

an•tag•o•nist
  adrenergic a.
  calcium a.

An•ta•zone

an•te•car•di•um

an•te•grade

an•ter•i•or

an•tero•grade

an•tero•in•fer•i•or

an•tero•lat•er•al

an•tero•me•di•al

an•tero•pos•ter•i•or

an•tero•sep•tal

an•tero•su•per•i•or

an•thra•cy•cline

an•thra•quin•one

an•ti•ad•re•ner•gic

an•ti•an•gi•nal

an•ti•ar•rhyth•mic

an•ti•ath•ero•gen•ic

an•ti•bi•ot•ic
  prophylactic a.

an•ti•body
  agglutinating a.
  anticardiolipin a.
  antiheart a.
  antimyosin a.
  antinuclear a's (ANA)
  cross-reacting a.
  cytotoxic B-cell a.
  monoclonal a's

an•ti•cho•les•ter•emic

an•ti•cho•les•te•rol•emic

an•ti•cho•lin•er•gic

an•ti•co•ag•u•lant
  lupus a.

an•ti•co•ag•u•la•tion

an•ti•de•pres•sant
  tricyclic a's

an•ti•di•uret•ic

an•ti-DNase B

an•ti•fib•ril•la•tory

an•ti•fi•bri•no•lyt•ic

an•ti•gen
  histocompatibility a's
  histocompatibility locus a.
  HLA a's
  human leukocyte a.
  human lymphocyte a.

an•ti•his•ta•mine

an•ti•hy•per•cho•les•ter•ol•emic

an•ti•hy•per•lipo•pro•tein•emic

an•ti•hy•per•ten•sive

an•ti•lipo•trop•ic

an•ti•lipo•trop•ism

an•ti•lym•pho•cyte

an•ti•mo•ny
  a. potassium tartrate
  a. sodium tartrate

an•ti•myo•sin

an•ti•psy•chot•ic

an•ti•strep•to•ly•sin O

an•ti•strep•to•zyme

an•ti•tachy•car•dia

an•ti•throm•bin
  a. I

an•ti•thy•mo•cyte

Ant•ley
  A.-Bixler syndrome

An•tu•rane

anu•lo•plas•ty

an•u•lus

AOO (atrial asynchronous) pace•maker

AOO (atrial asynchronous) pac•ing

aor•ta *pl.* aor•tae, aor•tas
  abdominal a.
  a. abdominalis
  a. ascendens
  ascending a.
  a. descendens
  descending a.
  descending thoracic a.
  dextropositioned a.
  interrupted a.
  overriding a.
  palpable a.
  a. sacrococcygea
  a. thoracalis
  thoracic a.

aor•ta *(continued)*
  a. thoracica
  ventral a.

aor•tal

aor•tal•gia

aor•tec•to•my

aor•tic

aor•tic arch syn•drome

aor•tic ar•ter•itis syn•drome

aor•ti•co•me•di•as•ti•nal

aor•ti•co•pul•mo•nary

aor•ti•co•re•nal

aor•tic throm•bo•em•bo•lism dis•ease

aor•ti•tis
  Döhle-Heller a.
  luetic a.
  nummular a.
  rheumatic a.
  syphilitic a.
  a. syphilitica

aor•to•bi•fem•o•ral

aor•to•ca•val

aor•to•cor•o•nary

aor•to•fem•o•ral

aor•to•gram

aor•tog•ra•phy
  retrograde a.
  translumbar a.

aor•to•il•i•ac

aor•top•a•thy

aor•to•plas•ty

aor•to•pul•mo•nary

aor•tor•rha•phy

aor•to•scle•ro•sis

aor•tot•o•my

APB
atrial premature beat

APC
atrial premature complex

Apert
A's syndrome

aper•tu•ra *pl.* aper•tu•rae
a. thoracis inferior
a. thoracis superior

ap•er•ture
inferior a. of thorax
superior a. of thorax
thoracic a., inferior
thoracic a., superior

apex *pl.* apex•es, api•ces
cardiac a.
a. cordis
a. of heart

apex•car•dio•gram
hyperdynamic a.

apex•car•di•og•ra•phy

ap•nea
sleep a.

apoA
apolipoprotein A

apo(a)
apolipoprotein (a)

Apo-Ac•et•a•zol•amide

Apo-Ami•trip•ty•line

Apo-Amoxi

Apo-Am•pi

Apo-Aten•o•lol

apoB
apolipoprotein B

apoC
apolipoprotein C

Apo-Car•ba•maz•e•pine

ap•o•ce•no•sis

Apo-Chlor•tha•li•done

Apo-Ci•met•i•dine

Apo-Cloxi

apoD
apolipoprotein D

Apo-Di•az•e•pam

Apo-Dil•ti•az

Apo-Di•py•rid•a•mole

apoE
apolipoprotein E

Apo-Eryth•ro

Apo-Flu•raz•e•pam

Apo-Fu•ro•sem•ide

Apo-Guan•eth•i•dine

Apo-Hy•dro

Apo-Imip•ra•mine

Apo-In•do•meth•a•cin

Apo-ISDN

apo•lipo•pro•tein
a. A
a. A-I
a. A-II
a. (a)
a. B
a. B-48
a. B-100
a. C
a. C-I
a. C-II
a. C-III
a. D
a. E
a. E2-4
thin line a.

Apo-Lor•a•ze•pam

Apo-Meth•yl•do•pa

Apo-Me•to•pro•lol

Apo-Me•tro•ni•da•zole

Apo-Ni•fed

Apo-Ox•az•e•pam

Apo-Phen•yl•bu•ta•zone

ap•o•plexy
 pancreatic a.

Apo-Pred•ni•sone

Apo-Pro•pran•o•lol

apo•pro•tein
 a. E

Apo-Sul•fa•meth•ox•a•zole

Apo-Sul•fa•trim

Apo-Sul•fin•py•ra•zone

Apo-Sul•in

Apo-Ti•mol

Apo-Tri•a•zo

Apo-Tri•mip

Apo-Ver•ap

ap•pa•rat•us *pl.* ap•pa•rat•us, ap•pa•rat•us•es
 Jaquet's a.
 vasomotor a.

ap•pen•dage
 atrial a.
 auricular a.
 right atrial a.

ap•pen•dec•to•my
 auricular a.

ap•pen•dix *pl.* ap•pen•di•ces, ap•pen•dix•es
 auricular a.

ap•proach

ap•prox•i•ma•tor
 Pilling Wolvek sternal a.
 rib a.
 sternal a.

Apres•o•line

apron
 lead a.

apro•ti•nin

aq•ua *pl.* aq•uae

Aqua•phyl•lin

Aq•ua•tag

Aq•ua•ten•sen

Ar
 argon

ara•chic acid

arach•i•date

ar•a•chid•ic acid

arach•i•don•ate

arach•i•don•ic acid

arach•no•dac•ty•ly

ARAD
 abnormal right axis deviation

Ar•a•len

Ar•a•mine

Aran•ti•us
 bodies of A.
 nodules of A.

ar•bo•ri•za•tion

ar•bo•vi•rus

arch
 a. of aorta
 aortic a's
 branchial a's
 cervical aortic a.
 double aortic a.
 jugular venous a.
 right aortic a.

ar•cus *pl.* ar•cus
 a. aortae
 corneal a.
 a. venosus juguli

ARDS
acute respiratory distress syndrome
adult respiratory distress syndrome

area *pl.* areae, areas
aortic a.
atrioventricular junctional a.
AV junctional a.
Bamberger's a.
body surface a.
a. of superficial cardiac dullness

ARF
acute rheumatic fever

Ar•fon•ad

ar•gi•nine
a. vasopressin

ar•gon

Ar•gyll Rob•ert•son
A.R. pupil

Arm-a-Med Iso•eth•a•rine

ar•rest
asystolic a.
atrial a.
bradyarrhythmic a.
cardiac a.
cardioplegic a.
cold cardioplegic a.
cold ischemic a.
deep hypothermia circulatory a.
heart a.
sinus a.
total circulatory a.
ventricular a.

Ar•rhi•gi
point of A.

ar•rhyth•mia
atrial a.
cardiac a.
continuous a.

ar•rhyth•mia *(continued)*
juvenile a.
lethal a.
malignant ventricular a.
nodal a.
nonphasic a.
nonrespiratory sinus a.
perpetual a.
phasic a.
reperfusion a.
respiratory a.
sinus a.
supraventricular a.
ventricular a.
ventricular ectopic a.

ar•rhyth•mic

ar•rhyth•mo•gen•e•sis

ar•rhyth•mo•gen•ic

ar•se•nic

ar•ter•ec•to•my

ar•te•ria *pl.* ar•te•riae
a. acetabuli
a. anonyma
a. aorta
a. axillaris
a. basilaris
a. brachialis
a. brachialis superficialis
arteriae bronchiales
arteriae caroticotympanicae
a. carotis communis
a. carotis externa
a. carotis interna
a. caudae pancreatis
a. cervicalis ascendens
a. cervicalis profunda
a. cervicalis superficialis
a. circumflexa anterior humeri
a. circumflexa femoris lateralis
a. circumflexa femoris medialis

ar•te•ria *(continued)*
a. circumflexa humeri anterior
a. circumflexa humeri posterior
a. circumflexa ilium profunda
a. circumflexa ilium superficialis
a. circumflexa posterior humeri
a. circumflexa scapulae
a. colica dextra
a. colica media
a. colica sinistra
a. collateralis media
a. collateralis radialis
a. collateralis ulnaris inferior
a. collateralis ulnaris superior
a. comitans nervi ischiadici
a. comitans nervi mediani
a. coronaria [cordis] dextra
a. coronaria dextra
a. coronaria [cordis] sinistra
a. coronaria sinistra
a. cystica
a. descendens genicularis
a. dorsalis scapularis
a. epigastrica inferior
a. epigastrica superficialis
a. epigastrica superior
a. femoralis
a. fibularis
arteriae gastricae breves
a. gastrica dextra
a. gastrica posterior
a. gastrica sinistra
a. gastroduodenalis
a. gastroepiploica dextra
a. gastroepiploica sinistra
a. gastro-omentalis dextra
a. gastro-omentalis sinistra
a. genus descendens

ar•te•ria *(continued)*
a. genus inferior lateralis
a. genus inferior medialis
a. genus media
a. genus superior lateralis
a. genus superior medialis
a. glutaea inferior
a. glutaea superior
a. glutea inferior
a. glutea superior
a. hepatica
a. hepatica communis
a. hepatica propria
a. hypogastrica
a. ileocolica
a. iliaca communis
a. iliaca externa
a. iliaca interna
a. iliolumbalis
a. inferior lateralis genus
a. inferior medialis genus
a. innominata
arteriae intercostales posteriores
a. intercostalis posterior prima
a. intercostalis posterior secunda
a. intercostalis suprema
arteriae interlobulares hepatis
arteriae interlobulares renis
a. interossea anterior
a. interossea communis
a. interossea dorsalis
a. interossea posterior
a. interossea recurrens
a. interossea volaris
arteriae intestinales
a. laryngea inferior
a. laryngea superior
a. lienalis
a. lobi caudati
arteriae lumbales
a. lusoria
a. lumbalis ima
a. mammaria interna

ar•te•ria *(continued)*
a. maxima Galeni
a. media genus
a. mediana
arteriae mediastinales anteriores
a. mesenterica inferior
a. mesenterica superior
a. musculophrenica
a. nutricia
a. nutricia fibulae
a. nutricia tibiae
arteriae nutriciae femoris
arteriae nutriciae humeri
a. nutriens fibulae
a. nutriens tibiae
arteriae nutrientes femoris
arteriae nutrientes humeri
a. obturatoria
a. obturatoria accessoria
a. occipitalis
a. pancreatica dorsalis
a. pancreatica inferior
a. pancreatica magna
arteriae pancreaticoduodenales inferiores
a. pancreaticoduodenalis superior anterior
a. pancreaticoduodenalis superior posterior
arteriae perforantes
a. pericardiacophrenica
a. peronea
arteriae phrenicae inferiores
arteriae phrenicae superiores
a. poplitea
a. profunda brachii
a. profunda femoris
a. pulmonalis
a. pulmonalis dextra
a. pulmonalis sinistra
a. radialis
a. recurrens radialis
a. recurrens tibialis anterior

ar•te•ria *(continued)*
a. recurrens tibialis posterior
a. recurrens ulnaris
arteriae renales
a. renalis
arteriae renis
arteriae retroduodenales
arteriae sacrales laterales
a. sacralis lateralis
a. sacralis media
a. sacralis mediana
a. scapularis descendens
a. scapularis dorsalis
a. segmenti anterioris
a. segmenti anterioris inferioris
a. segmenti anterioris superioris
a. segmenti inferioris
a. segmenti lateralis
a. segmenti medialis
a. segmenti posterioris
a. segmenti superioris
a. spinalis anterior
a. spinalis posterior
a. splenica
a. sternocleidomastoidea
a. subclavia
a. subcostalis
a. subscapularis
a. superior lateralis genus
a. superior medialis genus
a. supraduodenalis
arteriae suprarenales superiores
a. suprarenalis inferior
a. suprarenalis media
a. suprascapularis
arteriae surales
a. thoracica interna
a. thoracica lateralis
a. thoracica suprema
a. thoracoacromialis
a. thoracodorsalis
arteriae thymicae
a. thyreoidea ima
a. thyreoidea inferior

ar•te•ria *(continued)*
- a. thyreoidea superior
- a. thyroidea ima
- a. thyroidea inferior
- a. thyroidea superior
- a. tibialis anterior
- a. tibialis posterior
- a. transversa cervicis
- a. transversa colli
- a. transversa scapulae
- a. ulnaris
- a. umbilicalis
- a. vertebralis

ar•te•ri•al

ar•te•ri•ec•ta•sia

ar•te•ri•ec•ta•sis

ar•te•ri•ec•to•my

ar•te•ri•ec•to•pia

ar•te•rio•cap•il•lary

ar•te•rio•di•lat•ing

ar•te•rio•gram

ar•te•rio•graph

ar•te•ri•og•ra•phy
- Amplatz technique for coronary a.
- catheter a.
- coronary a.
- digital subtraction a.
- femoral a.
- Judkins coronary a.
- selective a.
- Sones technique for coronary a.
- two-dimensional a.

ar•te•rio•he•pat•ic dys•pla•sia syn•drome

ar•te•ri•o•la *pl.* ar•te•ri•o•lae

ar•te•ri•o•lar

ar•te•ri•ole

ar•te•rio•lith

ar•te•rio•li•tis

ar•te•ri•ol•o•gy

ar•te•ri•o•lop•a•thy

ar•te•rio•lo•scle•ro•sis

ar•te•rio•lo•scle•rot•ic

ar•te•rio•mo•tor

ar•te•rio•myo•ma•to•sis

ar•te•rio•ne•cro•sis

ar•te•ri•op•a•thy
- hypertensive a.
- plexogenic pulmonary a.
- thrombotic pulmonary a.

ar•te•rio•plas•ty

ar•te•rio•pres•sor

ar•te•ri•or•rha•phy

ar•te•ri•or•rhex•is

ar•te•rio•scle•ro•sis
- coronary a.
- hyaline a.
- hypertensive a.
- intimal a.
- medial a.
- Mönckeberg's a.
- a. obliterans
- peripheral a.
- presenile a.
- senile a.

ar•te•rio•scle•rot•ic

ar•te•ri•os•i•ty

ar•te•rio•spasm

ar•te•rio•spas•tic

ar•te•rio•ste•no•sis

ar•te•ri•os•teo•gen•e•sis

ar•te•ri•os•to•sis

ar•te•rio•strep•sis

ar•te•ri•ot•o•my
brachial a.

ar•te•ri•ot•o•ny

ar•te•ri•ous

ar•te•rio•ve•nous

ar•ter•itis *pl.* ar•ter•it•i•des
brachiocephalic a.
a. brachiocephalica
coronary a.
cranial a.
disseminated giant cell a.
giant cell a.
granulomatous a.
Horton's a.
localized visceral a.
necrotizing a.
a. nodosa
a. obliterans
renal a.
rheumatic a.
syphilitic a.
Takayasu's a.
temporal a.
tuberculous a.

ar•te•ry
aberrant a.
accessory a.
accompanying a. of ischiadic nerve
accompanying a. of median nerve
acetabular a.
a. of Adamkiewicz
anastomotic atrial a.
articular a., proper, of little head of fibula
atrial anastomotic a.
atrioventricular nodal a.
auricular a., left
auricular a., right
axillary a.
basilar a.
brachial a.
brachial a., deep
brachial a., superficial

ar•te•ry *(continued)*
brachiocephalic a.
bronchial a's
bronchial a's, anterior
capsular a., inferior
capsular a., middle
caroticotympanic a's
carotid a., common
carotid a., external
carotid a., internal
caudal a.
cephalic a.
cervical a., ascending
cervical a., deep
cervical a., superficial
cervical a., transverse
circumflex a., deep, internal
circumflex a., femoral, lateral
circumflex a., femoral, medial
circumflex a., humeral, anterior
circumflex a., humeral, posterior
circumflex a., iliac, deep
circumflex a., iliac, superficial
circumflex a. of scapula
coccygeal a.
Cohnheim's a.
colic a., left
colic a., middle
colic a., right
colic a., right, inferior
collateral a.
common femoral a.
collateral a., middle
collateral a., radial
collateral a., ulnar, inferior
collateral a., ulnar, superior
conal a.
conducting a's
conus a.
conus a., left

ar•te•ry *(continued)*
conus a., right
conus a., third
copper-wire a's
coronary a.
coronary a., descending, posterior
coronary a., left, of heart
coronary a., left, of stomach
coronary a., right, of heart
coronary a., right, of stomach
cystic a.
deltoid a.
diaphragmatic a's
diaphragmatic a's, superior
distributing a's
duodenal a's
elastic a's
emulgent a.
end a.
epigastric a., external
epigastric a., inferior
epigastric a., superficial
epigastric a., superior
esophageal a's, inferior
facial a.
femoral a.
femoral a., common
femoral a., deep
femoral a., superficial
fibular a.
gastric a., left
gastric a., left inferior
gastric a., posterior
gastric a., right
gastric a., right inferior
gastric a's, short
gastroduodenal a.
gastroepiploic a., left
gastroepiploic a., right
gastro-omental a., left
gastro-omental a., right
genicular a., descending
genicular a., inferior, lateral

ar•te•ry *(continued)*
genicular a., inferior, medial
genicular a., middle
genicular a., superior, lateral
genicular a., superior, medial
gluteal a., inferior
gluteal a., superior
great a's
hardening of a's
hepatic a., common
hepatic a., proper
a's of hybrid type
hypogastric a.
ileocolic a.
iliac a., anterior
iliac a., common
iliac a., external
iliac a., internal
iliac a., small
iliolumbar a.
infracostal a.
inguinal a's
innominate a.
intercostal a's, anterior
intercostal a., first posterior
intercostal a., highest
intercostal a's, posterior
intercostal a., second posterior
intercostal a., superior
interlobular a's of kidney
interlobular a's of liver
intermediate atrial a., left
intermediate atrial a., right
internal mammary a.
interosseous a., anterior
interosseous a., common
interosseous a., dorsal, of forearm
interosseous a., posterior, of forearm
interosseous a., recurrent
interosseous a., volar

ar•te•ry *(continued)*
interventricular a., anterior
interventricular septal a's, anterior
interventricular septal a's, posterior
intestinal a's
laryngeal a., inferior
laryngeal a., superior
left anterior descending a.
left circumflex a.
left main coronary a.
lumbar a's
lumbar a., fifth
lumbar a., lowest
major aortopulmonary collateral a.
mammary a., external
mammary a., internal
marginal a., left
marginal a., right
median a.
mediastinal a's, anterior
mediastinal a's, posterior
medullary a.
mesenteric a., inferior
mesenteric a., superior
a's of mixed type
muscular a's
musculophrenic a.
Neubauer's a.
nodal a.
noncoronary a.
nutrient a.
nutrient a's of femur
nutrient a. of fibula
nutrient a's of humerus
nutrient a's of kidney
nutrient a. of tibia
obturator a.
obturator a., accessory
occipital a.
pancreatic a., dorsal
pancreatic a., great
pancreatic a., inferior
pancreaticoduodenal a., anterior superior

ar•te•ry *(continued)*
pancreaticoduodenal a's, inferior
pancreaticoduodenal a., posterior superior
pelvic a., posterior
perforating a's
pericardiac a's, posterior
pericardiacophrenic a.
peroneal a.
peroneal a., perforating
phrenic a's, great
phrenic a's, inferior
phrenic a., superior
popliteal a.
proper articular a. of little head of fibula
pudendal a's, external
pudendal a., internal
pulmonary a.
pulmonary a., left
pulmonary a., right
pyloric a.
quadriceps a. of femur
radial a.
radial a., collateral
radiate a's of kidney
radicular a's
ranine a.
recurrent a., radial
recurrent a., tibial, anterior
recurrent a., tibial, posterior
recurrent a., ulnar
renal a.
renal a's
retrocostal a.
revehent a.
sacral a's, lateral
sacral a., median
sacrococcygeal a.
scapular a., descending
scapular a., dorsal
scapular a., transverse
sciatic a.
segmental a., anterior

ar•te•ry *(continued)*
segmental a., anterior inferior
segmental a., anterior superior
segmental a., inferior
segmental a., lateral
segmental a., medial
segmental a., posterior
segmental a., superior
septal a's, anterior
septal a's, posterior
sinoatrial nodal a.
sinuatrial nodal a.
sinus node a.
spinal a's
spinal a., anterior
spinal a., posterior
splenic a.
sternal a's, posterior
sternocleidomastoid a.
subclavian a.
subcostal a.
subscapular a.
supraduodenal a.
suprarenal a., aortic
suprarenal a., inferior
suprarenal a., middle
suprarenal a's, superior
sural a's
terminal a.
thoracic a., highest
thoracic a., internal
thoracic a., lateral
thoracicoacromial a.
thoracodorsal a.
thymic a's
thyroid a., inferior
thyroid a., lowest
thyroid a., superior
tibial a., anterior
tibial a., posterior
transverse cervical a.
transverse a. of neck
ulnar a.
ulnar collateral a., inferior
ulnar collateral a., superior

ar•te•ry *(continued)*
umbilical a.
venous a's
vertebral a.

ar•thri•tis *pl.* ar•thrit•i•des
Jaccoud's a.
rheumatoid a.

ar•ti•fact
flow a.
standardization a.
stimulus a.

ar•ti•fi•cial heart
air-driven a.h.
Jarvik 7 a.h.
total a.h.
Utah a.h.

Ar•vin

AS
ankylosing spondylitis
aortic stenosis

As
arsenic

Asa•san•tine

Asch•ner
A's phenomenon
A's reflex
A's sign
A's test
A.-Danini test

Asch•off
A's bodies
A's cells
A's node
A's nodules
node of A. and Tawara

as•ci•tes

as•cor•bic acid

ASD
atrial septal defect

Asen•din

ASH
asymmetrical septal hypertrophy

Ash•man
A's phenomenon

Ask
A.-Upmark kidney
A.-Upmark syndrome

As•ma•lix

ASO
antistreptolysin O

as•par•tate ami•no•trans•fer•ase

as•per•gil•lo•sis

As•per•gil•lus

as•phyg•mia

as•phyx•i•a•tion

as•pi•rate

as•pi•ra•tion

as•pi•rin
dipyridamole and a.
a., sodium bicarbonate, and citric acid

asple•nia

as•say
enzyme-linked immunosorbent a. (ELISA)

as•sess•ment
arterial graft a.
cardiac function a.
cardiovascular disability a.

AST
aspartate aminotransferase

as•the•nia
neurocirculatory a.

as•thma
bronchial a.

as•thma *(continued)*
cardiac a.
Elsner's a.
Heberden's a.
Rostan's a.

As•tra•morph

ASTZ
antistreptozyme

ASVIP (atrial synchronous ventricular inhibited) pace•maker

asyn•chro•nous

asyn•chro•ny

asyn•e•re•sis

asyn•er•gy

asys•to•le
atrial a.
mechanical a.
ventricular a.

asys•to•lia

asys•tol•ic

AT
atrial tachycardia

AT-III
antithrombin III

atax•ia
Friedreich's a.
hereditary a.
spastic a.
spinocerebellar a.

at•e•lec•ta•sis

aten•o•lol

ath•er•ec•to•my

ath•er•o•em•bo•lic

ath•ero•em•bo•lism

ath•ero•em•bo•lus *pl.* ath•ero•em•bo•li

ath•ero•gen•e•sis

ath•ero•gen•ic

ath•er•o•ma

ath•er•o•ma•to•sis

ath•er•o•ma•tous

ath•ero•scle•ro•sis
a. obliterans
premature a.

ath•ero•scle•rot•ic

Ati•van

ATP
adenosine triphosphate

ATPase
adenosinetriphosphatase

ATPP
activated partial thromboplastin time

atra•cu•rium bes•y•late

atre•sia
aortic a.
mitral a.
pulmonary a.
pulmonic a.
tricuspid a.

atri•al

atrio•com•mis•su•ro•pexy

atrio•hi•si•an

atrio•meg•a•ly

atrio•nec•tor

atrio•pep•ti•dase

atrio•pep•ti•gen

atrio•pep•tin

atrio•sep•to•pexy

atrio•sep•to•plas•ty

atri•ot•o•my
right a.

atrio•ven•tric•u•lar

atri•o•ven•tric•u•la•ris com•mu•nis

atri•um *pl.* atria
common a.
a. cordis
a. dextrum
left a.
a. pulmonale
pulmonary a.
right a.
single a.
a. sinistrum

At•ro•mid-S

at•ro•phy
peroneal muscular a.
red a.

at•ro•pine
a. methonitrate
a. methylnitrate
a. oxide hydrochloride
a. sulfate

A/T/S

at•tack
Adams-Stokes a.
anxiety a.
Stokes-Adams a.
transient ischemic a.

at•ten•u•a•tion

Au
gold (L. aurum)

Auen•brug•ger
A's sign

aug•men•tor

au•ri•cle
left a.
right a.

au•ric•u•la *pl.* au•ric•u•lae
atrial a.
a. atrialis
a. atrii
a. atrii dextri
a. atrii sinistri

au•ric•u•la *(continued)*
a. cordis
a. dextra
a. dextra cordis
a. sinistra
a. sinistra cordis

au•ric•u•lar

au•ric•u•lo•ven•tric•u•lar

aus•cul•tate

aus•cul•ta•tion
cardiac a.
direct a.
dynamic a.
immediate a.
Korányi's a.
mediate a.

aus•cul•ta•to•ry

aus•cul•to•plec•trum

aus•cul•to•scope

Aus•tin Flint
A.F. murmur
A.F. phenomenon

Aus•tra•lian Ther•a•peu•tic Tri•al

Auten•rieth
A. and Fink's method

au•to•ag•glu•ti•nin
cold a.

au•to•an•ti•bo•dy
cold a.

au•to•au•di•ble

au•tog•e•nous

au•to•hyp•no•sis

au•to•im•mu•ni•ty

au•to•in•fu•sion

au•tol•o•gous

au•to•ma•tic•i•ty
abnormal a.
altered a.
enhanced normal a.
triggered a.

au•to•nom•ic

au•to•reg•u•la•tion
heterometric a.
homeometric a.

au•to•trans•fu•sion

auxo•car•dia

AV
arteriovenous
atrioventricular

avas•cu•lar

avas•cu•lar•i•za•tion

AV block

Aven•tyl

averaging
signal a.

Av•i•tene

AV junc•tion•al

AVN
atrioventricular node

A wave

a wave

ax•il•lary

ax•il•lo•bi•fem•o•ral

ax•il•lo•fem•o•ral

ax•il•lo•pop•lit•e•al

ax•is *pl.* ax•es
arterial a., costocervical
celiac a.
a. deviation
dorsoventral a.
electrical a.
electrical a. of heart
a. of heart
instantaneous electrical a.

ax•is *(continued)*
lead a.
long a.
mean electrical a.
phlebostatic a.
QRS a.
thoracic a.
thyroid a.

ax•o•graph

Ayer•cil•lin

Ayges•tin

aza•thio•prine
a. sodium

Az•lin

az•lo•cil•lin

az•o•te•mia
prerenal a.

Azul•fi•dine

az•y•go•esoph•a•ge•al

az•y•go•me•di•as•ti•nal

B

B
    boron

Ba
    barium

Ba·bin·ski
    B's syndrome
    B.-Vaquez syndrome

Bach·mann
    B's bundle

ba·cil·lus *pl.* ba·cil·li

bac·i·tra·cin

Back·haus
    B. towel clamp

bac·ter·e·mia

Bac·te·roi·des
    B. oralis

Bac·to·cill

Bac·to·pen

Bac·trim

BAE
    bipolar atrial electrogram

baf·fle
    intra-atrial b.
    Mustard interatrial b.
    Senning intra-atrial b.

bag
    intestinal b.

Bai·ley
    B. rib contractor

Bain·bridge
    B. effect
    B. reflex

BAL
    bronchoalveolar lavage

bal·ance
    acid-base b.

bal·ance *(continued)*
    calcium b.
    fluid b.
    lactate b.

Bal·ke
    B. protocol
    B.-Ware protocol
    B.-Ware test

Bal·ler
    B.-Gerold syndrome

bal·lis·to·car·dio·gram

bal·lis·to·car·di·o·graph

bal·lis·to·car·di·og·ra·phy

bal·loon
    b. catheter
    intra-aortic b.
    b. pump

bal·loon·ing

bal·loon·ing mi·tral cusp syn·drome

Bam·ber·ger
    B's area
    B's sign

band
    A b.
    atrioventricular b.
    auriculoventricular b.
    contraction b.
    His' b.
    I b.
    Matas' b.
    moderator b.
    b. of Reil

band·ing
    pulmonary artery b.

Ban·ti
    B's syndrome

barb

Bar•bi•ta

bar•bi•tur•ate

Bard
B. Cardiopulmonary Support System
B.-Parker blade

Bar•det
B.-Biedl syndrome
Laurence-Moon-Biedl-B. syndrome

barium

Bar•ker
Keith-Wagener-B. classification

Bar•low
B. syndrome

baro•trau•ma

Bar•ré
Guillain-B. syndrome

Ba•sal•jel

base
b. of heart

base•line

ba•sis *pl.* ba•ses
b. cordis

Bas•sen
B.-Kornzweig syndrome

bath•mo•trop•ic

bathy•car•dia

Bat•son
B's plexus

bat•te•ry
BCX b.
bromine complex b.
Celsa b.
double-barrier wrap b.
dry b.
external b.
external pacemaker b.

bat•te•ry *(continued)*
internal b.
internal pacemaker b.
lithium anode b.
lithium–copper sulfide b.
lithium-iodine b.
lithium–lead sulfide b.
lithium–silver chromate b.
lithium–thionyl chloride b.
mercury-zinc b.
nickel-cadmium b.
nonchemical b.
nuclear b.
pacemaker b.
permanent b.
polyvinyl pyridine b.
rechargeable b.
temporary b.
zinc-mercury b.

Baum•gar•ten
Cruveilhier-B. murmur

Bayes
B. theorem

bayes•ian anal•y•sis

Bay•liss
B. theory

Baz•ett
B's formula

BBB
bundle branch block

BBBB
bilateral bundle branch block

BCX (bromine complex) bat•te•ry

Be
beryllium

Bé•brard
B's ligament

Beals
B. contractural arachnodactyly syndrome

beat
apex b.
atrial b.
atrial premature b.
atrioventricular junctional escape b.
blocked b.
capture b's
confusion b.
dropped b.
echo b.
ectopic b.
ectopic premature b.
escape b.
escaped b's
forced b.
fusion b.
junctional b.
paired b's
paired cardiac b's
premature b.
premature ventricular b.
reciprocal b's
sinus b.
sinus-conducted b.
ventricular b.
ventricular fusion b.
ventricular premature b.

Beau
B's disease
B's syndrome

Bea•ver
B. blade

Beck
B. miniature aorta clamp
B's triad
B. vascular clamp

Beck•er
B's cardiomyopathy
B's disease
B's dystrophy
B's muscular dystrophy

Beck•man
B. self-retaining retractor

Beck•with
B.-Wiedemann syndrome

bec•lo•meth•a•sone di•pro•pi•o•nate

bed
capillary b.
capillary exchange b.
vascular b.

be•hav•ior
type A b.
type B b.

Beh•çet
B's syndrome

be•ka•na•my•cin

Ben•a•dryl

ben•dro•flu•me•thi•a•zide

Bent•ley Oxy-State Me•ter

ben•zi•dine ox•i•dase

ben•zo•di•az•e•pine
b. hydrochloride

benz•thi•a•zide

ben•zyl•pen•i•cil•lin

bep•ri•dil

beri•beri
atrophic b.
dry b.
infantile b.
paralytic b.
ship b.
wet b.

beri•beri heart dis•ease

beri•ber•ic

Bern•heim
B's syndrome

Ber•noul•li
B's theorem

ber•yl•li•um

be•ta-ac•ti•nin

be•ta-ad•re•ner•gic

be•ta-adre•no•cep•tor
cardiac b.-a.

be•ta_2-ag•o•nist

be•ta-bloc•ker

be•ta-cho•les•ta•nol

Be•ta•loc

be•ta•meth•a•sone
b. acetate
b. benzoate
b. dipropionate
b. sodium phosphate
b. valerate

be•ta si•tos•ter•ol

be•ta throm•bo•glob•u•lin

be•thane•chol
b. chloride

be•than•i•dine sul•fate

Be•thune
B. rib shears

Bet•nel•an

Be•zold
B. reflex
B.-Jarisch reflex

BHE
bipolar His electrogram

Bi
bismuth

Bi•an•chi
B's nodules

bi•cam•er•al

bi•car•bo•nate
sodium b.

bi•car•bo•na•tu•ria

Bi•chat
B's membrane

Bi•cil•lin

bi•cus•pid

Bid•der
B's ganglia

Biedl
Bardet-B. syndrome
Laurence-B. syndrome
Laurence-Moon-B. syndrome
Laurence-Moon-B.-Bardet syndrome

Bi•fen•a•bid

bi•fur•ca•tio *pl.* bi•fur•ca•ti•o•nes
b. aortae
b. aortica
b. carotidis
b. trunci pulmonalis

bi•fur•ca•tion
b. of aorta
carotid b.
coronary b.
pulmonary b.
b. of pulmonary trunk

bi•fur•ca•tion•al

bi•gem•i•na

bi•gem•i•ny
atrial b.
nodal b.
ventricular b.

bi•lat•er•al

bile ac•id

Bili•vist

bil•low•ing mi•tral valve syn•drome

Bing
Taussig-B. syndrome
Taussig-B. type double outlet right ventricle

bio•avail•a•bil•i•ty

bio•de•te•ri•o•ra•tion

bio•im•plant

bio•ma•te•ri•al

Bio-Med•i•cus centrifugal pump

bio•pros•the•sis

bi•op•sy
endomyocardial b.
transvenous endomyocardial b.

bi•op•tome
Konno-Sakakibara b.
Stanford b.

Bio•tir•mone

Bio•tron•ik lead connector

bi•phas•ic

bi•plane

bi•po•lar

BIRA
bilateral intrapleural regional analgesia

bis•fe•ri•ous

Bish•op
B's sphygmoscope

bis•hy•droxy•cou•ma•rin

bis•muth
milk of b.
b. telluride

Bisp•ing
B. lead

bite
snake b.

bi•tol•ter•ol

bi•ven•tric•u•lar

Bix•ler
Antley-B. syndrome

Björk
B.-Shiley convexoconcave prosthetic valve

Björk *(continued)*
B.-Shiley monostrut prosthetic valve
B.-Shiley prosthetic valve

blade
Bard-Parker b.
Beaver b.
saw b.
sternal saw b.

Bla•lock
B. shunt
B.-Hanlon atrial septectomy
B.-Hanlon operation
B.-Taussig anastomosis
B.-Taussig operation
B.-Taussig shunt

Blas•to•my•ces

blas•to•my•co•sis

bleed•er

Blen•ox•ane

ble•o•my•cin
b. sulfate

bleph•a•ro•phi•mo•sis syn•drome

Blo•ca•dren

block
2:1 b.
anterior divisional b.
arborization b.
atrioventricular b.
2:1 atrioventricular b.
3:1 atrioventricular b.
atrioventricular heart b.
atrioventricular nodal b.
AV b.
1° AV b.
2° AV b.
3° AV b.
2:1 AV b.
3:1 AV b.
AV nodal b.
bifascicular b.

block *(continued)*
- bifascicular heart b.
- bilateral bundle branch b.
- bundle branch b.
- complete atrioventricular (AV) b.
- complete bundle branch b.
- complete heart b.
- conduction b.
- congenital complete AV b.
- congenital complete heart b.
- congenital heart b.
- divisional b.
- divisional heart b.
- entrance b.
- exit b.
- familial heart b.
- fascicular b.
- fascicular heart b.
- first degree atrioventricular (AV) b.
- first degree heart b.
- heart b.
- high degree atrioventricular (AV) b.
- high grade atrioventricular (AV) b.
- high threshold exit b.
- incomplete bundle branch b.
- incomplete heart b.
- intermittent atrioventricular (AV) b.
- interventricular b.
- intra-atrial b.
- intraventricular b.
- left anterior fascicular b.
- left bundle branch b.
- left posterior fascicular b.
- Mobitz b.
- Mobitz atrioventricular b.
- Mobitz second degree heart b.
- Mobitz type I b.
- Mobitz type I second degree heart b.
- Mobitz type II b.

block *(continued)*
- Mobitz type II second degree heart b.
- pacemaker-ventricular b.
- paroxysmal atrioventricular (AV) b.
- partial atrioventricular (AV) b.
- partial heart b.
- peri-infarction b.
- posterior divisional b.
- retrograde atrioventricular (AV) b.
- right bundle branch b.
- SA b.
- second degree atrioventricular (AV) b.
- second degree heart b.
- sinoatrial b.
- sinoatrial conduction b.
- sinoatrial exit b.
- sinoauricular b.
- sinus b.
- sinus exit b.
- third degree atrioventricular (AV) b.
- third degree heart b.
- trifascicular b.
- type I atrioventricular nodal b.
- type I second degree atrioventricular b.
- type I second degree AV b.
- type I Wenckebach AV nodal b.
- type II atrioventricular nodal b.
- type II second degree b.
- type II second degree AV b.
- unidirectional b.
- unspecified intraventricular b.
- Wenckebach b.
- Wenckebach exit b.

block•ade
- β-adrenergic b.

block•ade *(continued)*
beta-b.
beta-adrenergic b.
beta-adrenoceptor b.
conduction b.
major conduction b.

blocker
α-adrenergic b.
β-adrenergic b.
adrenoceptor b.
alpha-adrenergic b.
alpha-adrenoceptor b.
beta b.
beta-adrenergic b.
beta-adrenoceptor b.
calcium b.
calcium channel b.
channel b.
cobra venom factor b.
ganglionic b.
muscarinic cholinergic b.
slow channel b.

blood
b. clot
b. count
b. culture
b. dyscrasia
b. flow
b. gases
mixed venous b.
b. pressure
b. volume

blood pres•sure

Bloor
B., Pelkan, and Allen's method

blue toe syn•drome

BMI
body mass index

B-mode ul•tra•so•nog•ra•phy

body
aortic b.
b's of Arantius
asbestos b's

body *(continued)*
asbestosis b's
Aschoff b's
bamboo b's
Bracht-Wächter b's
carotid b.
central fibrous b. of heart
jugulotympanic b.
para-aortic b's
supracardial b's
tympanic b.
vagal b.
Zuckerkandl's b's

Bo•ga•lu•sa Heart Study

BOH
bundle of His

BOL
beginning of (battery) life

bo•lom•e•ter

bol•ster

bo•lus

boot
silicone rubber b.

bor•der
b. of oval fossa
right b. of heart

Borg
B. scale

bo•ron

Bo•tal•lo
ligament of B.

bot•tle
chest drainage b.
drainage b.

Bouil•laud
B's sign
B's syndrome

Bou•ve•ret
B's disease
B's syndrome

bow
 cupid's b.

Bow•ditch
 B's law
 B. staircase phenomenon

Boz•zo•lo
 B's sign

BP
 blood pressure

BPL
 bronchopulmonary lavage

bpm
 beats per minute

Br
 bromine

bra•chi•al

Brach•mann
 B.-de Lange syndrome

Bracht
 B.-Wächter bodies
 B.-Wächter lesion

brachy•dac•ty•ly-sphe•ro•pha•kia syn•drome

Brad•bury
 B.-Eggleston syndrome

brady•ar•rhyth•mia

brady•car•dia
 Branham's b.
 central b.
 essential b.
 nodal b.
 postinfective b.
 sinoatrial b.
 sinus b.
 vagal b.
 ventricular b.

brady•car•di•ac

brady•car•dia-tachy•car•dia syn•drome

brady•car•dic

brady•crot•ic

brady•di•as•to•le

brady•dys•rhyth•mia

brady•ki•nin

brady•rhyth•mia

brady•sphyg•mia

brady•tachy•car•dia

branch
 bundle b.
 left bundle b.
 right bundle b.
 superior b.

Bran•ham
 B's bradycardia
 B's sign
 Nicoladoni-B. sign

Braun•wald
 B. sign

breast
 thrush b.

breath•ing
 intermittent positive pressure b.

Bre•thaire

Breth•ine

Bre•tyl•ate

bre•tyl•i•um to•sy•late

Bre•tyl•ol

Brevi•bloc

Bric•a•nyl

Brick•ner
 B's sign

bridge
 arteriolovenular b.
 Gaskell's b.
 Purkinje b.

bridg•ing
    myocardial b.

Broad•bent
    B's inverted sign
    B's sign

Brock
    B's infundibulectomy
    B's operation
    B's valvotomy

Brock•en•brough
    B's sign
    B. transseptal catheter

bro•mine

bro•mo•crip•tine

bron•chi•al

bron•chi•ec•ta•sis

bron•chi•tis
    chronic b.

bron•cho•con•stric•tion

bron•cho•con•stric•tor

bron•cho•di•la•tor

Bron•ko•dyl

Bron•ko•sol

Brown
    B. and Sharp (B&S) gauge
    Hines and B. test

Brown•lee
    B. code

Bruce
    B. protocol
    B. treadmill protocol
    modified B. protocol

Bru•cel•la

bru•cel•lo•sis

bruisse•ment

bruit
    aneurysmal b.
    b. de canon

bruit *(continued)*
    b. de choc
    b. de claquement
    b. de craquement
    b. de cuir neuf
    b. de diable
    false b.
    b. de froissement
    b. de frolement
    b. de frottement
    b. de galop
    b. de lime
    b. de moulin
    b. de parchemin
    b. de piaulement
    b. de rape
    b. de rappel
    b. de Roger
    Roger's b.
    b. de scie
    b. de soufflet
    systolic b.
    b. de tabourka
    b. de tambour

Brush•field
    B's spots

BSA
    body surface area

B&S (Brown and Sharp) gauge

BS (Björk-Shiley) pros•thet•ic valve

bu•car•dia

bud
    vascular b.

bud•ding

Buer•ger
    B's disease
    B's symptom
    Winiwater-B. disease

bulb
    b. of aorta
    b. of jugular vein, inferior
    b. of jugular vein, superior

bul•bo•atri•al

bul•bo•spi•ral

bul•bus *pl.* bul•bi
b. aortae
b. caroticus
b. cordis
b. inferior venae jugularis
b. superior venae jugularis
b. venae jugularis inferior
b. venae jugularis superior

bulge
diastolic b.

bu•met•a•nide

Bu•mex

BUN
blood urea nitrogen

bun•dle
atrioventricular b.
AV b.
Bachmann's b.
common b.
common b. of His
conduction b.
His b.
b. of His
Keith's b.
Kent's b.
Kent-His b.
main b.
sinoatrial b.
b. of Stanley Kent
Thorel's b.

bun•dle branch
b.b. block
left b.b.
b.b. reentry
right b.b.

bu•piv•a•caine hy•dro•chlo•ride

bu•pre•nor•phine
b. diazepam

bu•pro•pi•on hy•dro•chlo•ride

Bur•chard
Liebermann-B. reaction
Liebermann-B. test

Bur•ger
B's scalene triangle

Bu•row
B's vein

bu•sul•fan

Bu•ta•tab

Bu•ta•zol•i•din

Bu•ta•zone

but•ton
skin b.
velour skin b.

but•ton•hole
mitral b.

bu•ty•ryl

by•pass
aortobifemoral b.
aortocoronary b.
aortofemoral b.
aortofemoral b., thoracic
aortoiliac b.
axillobifemoral b.
axillofemoral b.
axillopopliteal b.
cardiopulmonary b.
coronary b.
coronary artery b.
EC/IC b.
extra-anatomic b.
extracranial/intracranial (EC/IC) b.
femoral crossover b.
femorofemoral b.
femorofemoropopliteal b.
femoropopliteal b.
heart-lung b.
hypothermic cardiopulmonary b.

by•pass *(continued)*
- left heart b.
- partial b.
- partial cardiopulmonary b.
- partial ileal b.

by•pass *(continued)*
- pulsatile cardiopulmonary b.
- right heart b.
- total cardiopulmonary b.

C

C
carbon
coulomb

C_L
pulmonary compliance

Ca
calcium

CAB
coronary artery bypass

CABG
coronary artery bypass graft

ca•ble
alligator pacing c.
fibrillator c.
grounding c.
pacing c.

ca•chex•ia
cardiac c.

caco•rhyth•mic

CAD
coronary artery disease

ca•dence
sinus c.

cad•mi•um
c. sulfide

caf•feine

cage

Cal•an

cal•ci•fi•ca•tion
arterial c.
coronary c.
metastatic c.
Mönckeberg's c.
pericardial c.

Cal•ci•le•an

cal•ci•no•sis

Cal•ci•par•ine

cal•ci•to•nin

cal•ci•um
c. channel
c. chloride
c. gluceptate
c. gluconate

cal•cu•lus *pl.* cal•cu•li
cholesterol c.

cam•era *pl.* cam•eras, cam•erae
Anger c.
Anger gamma c.
Anger scintillation c.
gamma c.
gamma scintillation c.
multicrystal scintillation c.
multiple crystal gamma c.
scintillation c.
single crystal scintillation c.
single crystal gamma c.

Cam•mann
C's stethoscope

Cam•py•lo•bac•ter

Can•a•da
C.-Cronkhite syndrome

Ca•na•di•an Car•dio•vas•cu•lar So•ci•e•ty

ca•nal
common atrioventricular c.
persistent common atrioventricular c.
Theile's c.
Verneuil's c's

Can•di•da

can•di•di•a•sis
endocardial c.

can•nu•la
aortic c.
aortic cardioplegic c.
atrial c.
coronary perfusion c.
femoral c.
left ventricular c.
vena cava c.
venous c.

can•nu•late

can•nu•la•tion
percutaneous right heart c.

can•ren•one

cap
lead pin c.

ca•pac•i•tance
coronary c.

ca•pac•i•tor

ca•pac•i•ty
aerobic c.
battery c.
maximal work c.
oxygen c.
pulmonary diffusing c.
vital c.

cap•il•lary
arterial c's
Meigs' c's
sinusoidal c.
venous c's

Cap•o•ten

Cap•o•zide

cap•ric acid

cap•ri•zant

ca•pro•ic acid

ca•pryl•ic acid

cap•su•la *pl.* cap•su•lae
c. cordis

cap•sule
c. of heart
pulse generator c.

cap•to•pril

cap•ture
cardiac c.

car•ba•chol

car•ba•maz•e•pine

car•ben•i•cil•lin
c. disodium
c. indanyl sodium
c. phenyl sodium
c. potassium
c. sodium

Car•bo•lith

car•bo•meth•oxy•iso•pro•pyl iso•ni•trile

car•bon
c. 11
c. dioxide
c. monoxide
c. palmitate
pyrolytic c.
vitreous c.

car•bon•ic an•hy•drase

car•ci•noid

car•ci•noid syn•drome

car•ci•no•ma *pl.* car•ci•no•mas, car•ci•no•ma•ta
atrial c.
medullary c.

Car•da•rel•li
C's sign

Car•dene

car•di•ac
c. alternans
c. anomalies
c. apex
c. arrest
c. arrhythmia

car•di•ac *(continued)*
c. asthma
c. auscultation
c. balloon pump
c. cachexia
c. capture
c. catheter
c. catheterization
c. cell
c. chamber
c. conduction
c. conduction system
c. contractility
c. contraction
c. contusion
c. cough
c. cycle
c. death
c. decomposition
c. digital fluoroscopy
c. dyspnea
c. electrophysiology
c. enlargement
c. enzymes
c. failure
c. function
c. function assessment
c. glycoside
c. hypertrophy
c. impulse
c. index
c. ischemia
c. lung
c. malformation
c. mapping
c. metabolism
c. murmur
c. muscle
c. myosin
c. nerves
c. output
c. output curve
c. output index
c. pacemaker
c. pacing
c. pacing system
c. perforation
c. performance

car•di•ac *(continued)*
c. pulsation
c. rehabilitation
c. reserve
c. respiratory reflex
c. resting potential
c. resuscitation
c. rhythm
c. risk index
c. roentgenography
c. rupture
c. scintigraphy
c. shunt
c. sidedness
c. silhouette
c. standstill
c. stiffness
c. surgery
c. syncope
c. tamponade
c. thrombus
c. transmural pressure
c. transplant
c. transplantation
c. tumor
c. valve
c. volume
c. wall thickening

car•di•ac-limb syn•drome

car•di•al•gia

car•di•ant

car•di•asth•ma

car•di•ec•ta•sis

Car•di•late

Car•dio-500

car•dio•ac•cel•er•a•tor

car•dio•ac•tive

car•dio•an•gi•og•ra•phy
radionuclide c.

car•dio•an•gi•ol•o•gy

car•dio•aor•tic

car•dio•ar•te•ri•al

Car•di•o•bac•te•ri•um
C. hominis

car•dio•cai•ro•graph

car•dio•cele

car•dio•cen•te•sis

car•dio•cir•cu•la•tory

car•dio•cir•rho•sis

car•dio•cyte

car•dio•di•a•phrag•mat•ic

car•dio•di•la•tin

car•dio•di•la•tor

car•dio•na•trin

car•dio•dy•nam•ics

car•di•odyn•ia

Car•dio•Gen-82

car•dio•gen•e•sis

car•dio•ge•net•ic

car•di•o•gen•ic

car•dio•gram
apex c.
esophageal c.
negative c.
precordial c.
vector c.

car•dio•graph

car•dio•graph•ic

car•di•og•ra•phy
apex c.
nuclear c.
radionuclide c.
ultrasonic c.
vector c.

Car•dio-Green

car•dio•he•pat•ic

car•dio•hep•a•to•meg•a•ly

car•di•oid

car•dio•in•hib•i•to•ry

car•dio•ki•net•ic

car•dio•ky•mo•graph•ic

car•dio•ky•mog•ra•phy

car•dio•lith

car•di•ol•o•gist

car•di•ol•o•gy
nuclear c.

car•di•ol•y•sis

car•dio•ma•la•cia

Car•dio Max

car•dio•me•ga•lia
c. glycogenica circumscripta
c. glycogenica diffusa

car•dio•meg•a•ly
glycogenic c.
idiopathic c.

car•dio•mel•a•no•sis

car•di•om•e•ter

car•di•om•e•try

car•dio•mo•til•i•ty

car•dio•myo•li•po•sis

car•dio•my•op•a•thy
African c.
alcoholic c.
apical hypertrophic c.
Becker's c.
beer-drinker's c.
chronic congestive c.
cobalt c.
congestive c.
dilated c.
familial c.
familial hypertrophic obstructive c.
fatty c.
genetic hypertrophic c.

car•dio•my•op•a•thy *(continued)*
- hypertrophic c.
- hypertrophic obstructive c.
- idiopathic dilated c.
- infiltrative c.
- ischemic c.
- nephropathic c.
- nonischemic c.
- nonobstructive hypertrophic c.
- obstructive hypertrophic c.
- pediatric c.
- peripartum c.
- postpartum c.
- primary c.
- primary congestive c.
- restrictive c.
- secondary c.
- thyrotoxic c.
- toxic c.

car•dio•myo•pexy

car•dio•ne•cro•sis

car•dio•nec•tor

car•dio•neph•ric

car•dio•neu•ral

car•dio•neu•rop•a•thy

car•dio-omen•to•pexy

car•dio•pal•u•dism

car•dio•path

car•dio•path•ia

car•dio•path•ic

car•di•op•a•thy
- infarctoid c.

car•dio•peri•car•dio•pexy

car•dio•peri•car•di•tis

car•dio•pho•bia

car•dio•phre•nia

car•dio•ple•gia
- cold c.

car•dio•ple•gia *(continued)*
- cold potassium c.

car•dio•ple•gic

car•dio•pneu•mat•ic

car•dio•pneu•mo•graph

car•dio•pneu•mono•pexy

car•dio•pro•tec•tive

car•di•op•to•sia

car•di•op•to•sis

car•dio•pul•mo•nary

car•dio•pul•mon•ic

car•dio•re•nal

car•di•or•rha•phy

car•di•or•rhex•is

car•dio•scle•ro•sis

car•dio•scope

car•dio•se•lec•tive

car•dio•se•lec•tiv•i•ty

car•dio•sphyg•mo•gram

car•dio•sphyg•mo•graph

car•dio•spleno•pexy

car•dio•ta•chom•e•ter

car•dio•ta•chom•e•try

car•dio•ther•a•py

car•dio•thy•ro•tox•ic

car•dio•to•co•graph

car•dio•to•cog•ra•phy

car•di•ot•o•my

car•dio•ton•ic

car•dio•to•pog•ra•phy

car•dio•to•pom•e•try

car•dio•tox•ic

car•dio•tox•ic•i•ty

car•dio•trop•ic

car•dio•val•vu•lar

car•dio•val•vu•li•tis

car•dio•val•vu•lo•tome

car•di•o•val•vu•lot•o•my

car•dio•vas•cu•lar

car•dio•vas•cu•lar-re•nal

car•dio•vas•ol•o•gy

car•dio•vec•tor•gra•phy

car•dio•ver•sion
- direct-current (DC) c.
- electrical c.
- internal epicardial c.
- transthoracic c.

car•dio•vert

car•dio•ver•ter

car•dio•ver•ter-de•fib•ril•la•tor
- automatic c.-d.
- automatic implantable c.-d.
- fully implantable c.-d.
- implantable c.-d.

car•dio•vi•rus

car•di•tis
- acute rheumatic c.
- maternal acute rheumatic c.
- rheumatic c.
- streptococcal c.
- verrucous c.

Car•di•zem

care
- coronary c.
- critical c.
- intensive c.
- managed c.

Car•ey Coombs
- C.C. murmur

ca•rot•id

ca•rot•i•dyn•ia

ca•rot•odyn•ia

Car•pen•ter
- C. syndrome

Car•pen•tier
- C. combined sternal-atrial retractor
- C. ring
- C. tricuspid obturator
- C. tricuspid ring
- C.-Edwards valve

car•te•o•lol hy•dro•chlo•ride

Car•trol

Car•va•llo
- C's sign
- Rivero-C. sign

cas•cade
- arachidonic acid c.
- coagulation c.

cas•ing
- Silastic c.

CASS
- Coronary Artery Surgery Study

cast

Cas•ta•ne•da
- C. anastomosis clamp
- C. multipurpose clamp

Cas•tel•li•no
- C's sign

CAT
- computerized axial tomography

cata•crot•ic

ca•tac•ro•tism

cata•di•crot•ic

cata•di•cro•tism

Cat•a•pres

cata•tri•crot•ic

cata•tri•cro•tism

cat•e•chol•amine

cat-eye syn•drome

cat•gut
  chromic c.

cath•e•ter
  c. adapter
  Amplatz coronary c.
  Angiocath c.
  angiographic c.
  arteriography c.
  atherectomy c.
  balloon c.
  balloon embolectomy c.
  balloon-tipped c.
  balloon-tipped flow-directed c.
  balloon-tipped thermodilution c.
  Brockenbrough transseptal c.
  cardiac c.
  central venous c.
  coronary dilatation c.
  Cournand c.
  dilatation c.
  double-lumen c.
  embolectomy c.
  femoral-internal mammary artery c.
  floating c.
  flow-directed c.
  fluid-filled c.
  Fogarty c.
  Fogarty balloon c.
  Foley c.
  French c.
  French-Robinson c.
  Gensini coronary arteriography c.
  Goodale-Lubin c.
  Gruentzig c.
  Gruentzig balloon c.

cath•e•ter *(continued)*
  guiding c.
  Hartzler LPS c.
  indwelling c.
  intra-aortic balloon c.
  intracardiac monitoring c.
  intravascular c.
  intravenous c.
  Judkins coronary c.
  Judkins left coronary c.
  Judkins left coronary arteriography c.
  Judkins pigtail left ventriculography c.
  Judkins right coronary c.
  Judkins right coronary arteriography c.
  left heart c.
  left ventricular c.
  left ventricular sump c.
  manometer-tipped c.
  micromanometer c.
  multipurpose c.
  nonpreformed c.
  NoProfile balloon c.
  Nycore-pigtail c.
  Olbert balloon c.
  Oximetrix fiberoptic pulmonary artery c.
  pacing c.
  pigtail c.
  plastic c.
  preformed c.
  pulmonary artery c.
  quadruple lumen c.
  radial artery c.
  reperfusion c.
  right heart c.
  Simpson atherectomy c.
  Simpson-Robert c.
  snare c.
  Sones coronary c.
  suction c.
  sump c.
  Swan-Ganz c.
  Swan-Ganz monitoring c.
  Teflon c.
  temperature-sensitive c.

cath•e•ter *(continued)*
thermodilution c.
c. tip
transluminal c.
triple lumen c.

cath•e•ter•iza•tion
cardiac c.
combined c.
hepatic vein c.
interventional cardiac c.
left heart c.
percutaneous arterial c.
retrograde c.
retrograde arterial c.
right heart c.
transseptal left-heart c.

cath•e•ter-mi•cro•phone
cardiac c.-m.

cath•ode
iodine c.
silver chromate c.
tip-stimulating c.

cau•dal

cau•ter•ize

cau•tery
electric c.

ca•va

ca•val

CAVB
complete atrioventricular block

cav•i•tas *pl.* cav•i•ta•tes
c. pericardialis
c. thoracis

ca•vi•tis

cav•i•ty
interatrial c.
intraventricular c.
mediastinal c., anterior
mediastinal c., middle
mediastinal c., posterior
mediastinal c., superior

cav•i•ty *(continued)*
pectoral c.
pericardial c.
thoracic c.

ca•vo•atri•al

ca•vog•ra•phy

ca•vo•pul•mo•nary

CBC
complete blood count

CBF
cerebral blood flow
coronary blood flow

cc
cubic centimeter

CCU
coronary care unit

Cd
cadmium

Ce•di•lan•id-D

Ce•do•card

cef•a•drox•il

Cef•a•dyl

Cef•a•nex

ce•faz•o•lin
c. sodium

Ceg•ka
C's sign

Ce•les•tone

cell
alpha-emitting nuclear power c.
Anichkov's c.
Aschoff's c's
atrial myocardial c.
automatic c.
battery c.
BCX power c.
beta-voltaic power c.
biofuel c.

cell *(continued)*
- biogalvanic c.
- biogalvanic hybrid fuel power c.
- bromine complex power c.
- cardiac c.
- clear c's
- double anode power c.
- double-barrier wrap power c.
- electrochemical c.
- endothelial c.
- excitable c.
- foam c's
- glomerular c.
- glomus c.
- heart-disease c's
- heart-failure c's
- heart-lesion c's
- Hurler c.
- lithium anode power c.
- lithium-bromine power c.
- lithium–copper sulfide power c.
- lithium-iodine power c.
- lithium–lead iodide power c.
- lithium–lead sulfide power c.
- lithium–manganese dioxide power c.
- lithium–silver chromate power c.
- lithium–thionyl chloride power c.
- lithium–titanium disulfide power c.
- littoral c's
- macrophage c.
- mast c.
- mercury-zinc power c.
- myointimal c.
- natural killer c.
- nickel-cadmium power c.
- NK c's
- nodal c.
- nonpacemaker c.
- nuclear power c.

cell *(continued)*
- P c.
- pacemaker c.
- pericapillary c's
- perivascular c's
- plutonium power c.
- polyvinyl pyridine power c.
- power c.
- promethium power c.
- proximal tubular c.
- Purkinje's c's
- rechargeable power c.
- red c.
- red blood c.
- Rouget c's
- SAFT power c.
- self-excitatory c.
- self-excitatory cardiac c.
- silver-mercury–silver-zinc power c.
- sinus nodal c.
- smooth muscle c.
- spider c.
- stave c's
- strap c.
- T c's
- technetium 99m–labeled red blood c.
- tennis racquet c.
- thermoelectric power c.
- transitional c.
- vasofactive c's
- vasoformative c's
- white c.
- white blood c.

cel•lu•lose
- oxidized c.

ce•lo•phle•bi•tis

Cel•sa
- C. battery
- C. power cell

cen•ter
- vasomotor c's

ceph•a•lad

ceph•a•lex•in
c. hydrochloride

ce•phal•ic

ceph•a•lin

ceph•a•li•za•tion
c. of pulmonary blood flow

ceph•a•lo•spo•rin

ceph•a•lo•thin
c. sodium

ceph•a•pi•rin
c. sodium

ceph•ra•dine

Ce•por•a•cin

Ce•por•ex

ce•ram•ic

cer•a•mide
c. trihexoside

cer•e•bro•car•di•ac

cer•e•bro•vas•cu•lar

Cer•e•span

Ce•ru•bi•dine

C.E.S.

ce•si•um

Cha•gas
C. disease

chal•lenge
standarized fluid c.

cham•ber
cardiac c.
c's of the heart
left heart c's
right heart c's
systemic pumping c.

change
reciprocal c's

chan•nel
calcium c.

chan•nel *(continued)*
central c.
fast c.
fast sodium c.
marker c.
membrane c.
receptor-operated c.
slow c.
slow sodium c.
sodium c.
thoroughfare c.
voltage-dependent c.

Char•cot
C's syndrome
C.-Marie-Tooth disease

Char•dack
C.-Greatbach pacemaker

CHARGE as•so•ci•a•tion

CHD
congenital heart disease
congestive heart disease
coronary heart disease

che•mo•ther•a•py

che•mo•tox•in

che•no•de•oxy•cho•late

che•no•de•oxy•cho•lic acid

che•no•de•oxy•cho•lyl•gly•cine

che•no•de•oxy•cho•lyl•tau•rine

Cher•a•gan W/TMP

chest
pigeon c.
shield c.

Cheyne
C.-Stokes respiration

CHF
congestive heart failure

Chi•a•ri
C's network

Chi•a•ri *(continued)*
C's reticulum

CHILD syn•drome

chi•mer•ism
allogeneic c.

Chla•myd•ia
C. psittaci
C. trachomatis

chlo•ride
thallous c. Tl 201
thionyl c.

chlo•rine

chlo•ro•quine
c. diphosphate
c. hydrochloride
c. phosphate

chlo•ro•thi•a•zide
c. sodium

chlor•phen•ir•amine
c. maleate

Chlor•prom•a•nyl

chlor•prom•a•zine
c. hydrochloride

chlor•thal•i•done

cho•la•ic acid

cho•lan•ic acid

cho•late

Cho•les•ta•byl

cho•les•tane

cho•les•ta•ne•tri•ol

cho•les•ta•nol
beta-c.

cho•les•ter•emia

cho•les•ter•in

cho•les•ter•in•emia

cho•les•tero•gen•e•sis

cho•les•ter•ol
high density c.

cho•les•ter•ol acyl•trans•fer•ase

Cho•les•ter•ol Con•sen•sus Con•fer•ence

cho•les•ter•ol des•mol•ase

cho•les•ter•ol•emia

cho•les•ter•ol•er•e•sis

cho•les•ter•ol mono•oxy•gen•ase (side-chain cleav•ing)

cho•les•ter•olo•poi•e•sis

cho•les•ter•yl

cho•les•ter•yl es•ter stor•age dis•ease

cho•les•ty•ra•mine res•in

cho•lic acid

cho•lin•er•gic

cho•lin•es•ter•ase

cho•li•no•mi•met•ics
muscarinic c.

Cho•lox•in

Choly•bar

cho•lyl•gly•cine

cho•lyl•tau•rine

chor•da *pl.* chor•dae
chordae tendineae
c. tendineae cordis

cho•rea
c. gravidarum
mitral valve c.
non-ejection systolic c.
Sydenham's c.

Chot•zen
C's syndrome
Saethre-C. syndrome

Christ•mas tree lead

chro•mi•um

Chro•mo•bac•ter

Chro•mo•spo•ri•num

chron•o•sphyg•mo•graph

chron•o•trop•ic

chron•o•trop•ism

Churg
C.-Strauss syndrome

chy•lo•mi•cron *pl.* chyl•lo•mi•crons, chy•lo•mi•cra
c. remnant

chy•lo•mi•cro•ne•mia

chy•lo•peri•car•di•tis

chy•lo•peri•car•di•um
idiopathic c.

CI
cardiac index

Ci
curie

Ciba•lith

Ci•do•my•cin

cil•a•sta•tin

ci•met•i•dine
c. hydrochloride

cine•an•gio•car•diog•ra•phy
radionuclide c.

cine•an•gio•gram

cine•an•gio•graph

cine•an•gi•og•ra•phy
coronary c.
radionuclide c.

cine•flu•o•rog•ra•phy

cine•flu•o•ros•co•py

Cine•loop digital image review

cine•ma•tog•ra•phy

cine•ma•to•ra•di•og•ra•phy

cine•phle•bog•ra•phy

cine•ra•di•og•ra•phy

cine•roent•geno•flu•o•rog•ra•phy

cine•roent•gen•og•ra•phy
arterial c.
Robinson's c.
vascular c.

cir•cuit
asynchronous c.
demand c.
hybrid c.
IC c.
incomplete c.
inductance-capacitance (IC) c.
integrated c.
macroreentrant c.
microreentrant c.
miniature c.
pulse generator c.
quartz crystal c.
RC c.
reentrant c.
reentry c.
resistance-capacitance c.
sensing c.
short c.
timing c.

cir•cu•la•tion
assisted c.
collateral c.
collateral parietal c.
compensatory c.
coronary c.
coronary collateral c.
derivative c.
extracorporeal c.
fetal c.
greater c.
lesser c.
peripheral c.
persistent fetal c.
portal c.
pulmonary c.

cir•cu•la•tion *(continued)*
- sinusoidal c.
- systemic c.
- thebesian c.
- c. time

cir•cu•la•tor

cir•cu•la•to•ry

cir•cu•lus *pl.* cir•cu•li
- c. arteriosus
- c. articularis vasculosus
- c. vasculosus

cir•cum•vas•cu•lar

cir•rho•sis
- hepatic c.
- c. of liver

cir•soid

cis•pla•tin

cis•ter•na *pl.* cis•ter•nae
- subsarcolemmal cisternae

cit•rate

cit•ric acid
- aspirin, sodium bicarbonate, and c.a.

Cit•ro•bac•ter

CK
- creatine kinase

CK-MB
- myocardial muscle creatine kinase isozyme

CK-MM
- skeletal muscle creatine kinase isozyme

Cl
- chlorine

clamp
- Allis c.
- anastomosis c.
- angled vascular c.
- aorta c.
- aortic cross c.

clamp *(continued)*
- Backhaus towel c.
- Beck miniature aorta c.
- Beck vascular c.
- bronchus c.
- bulldog c.
- cardiovascular c.
- Castaneda anastomosis c.
- Castaneda multipurpose c.
- coarctation c.
- Cooley coarctation c.
- Cooley multipurpose c.
- Cooley partially occluding vascular c.
- Cooley patent ductus c.
- Cooley pediatric c.
- Cooley vascular c.
- Cooley vena cava c.
- Crafoord c.
- Crafoord coarctation c.
- Crile's c.
- curved c.
- curved mosquito c.
- curved vascular c.
- DeBakey bulldog c.
- DeBakey coarctation c.
- DeBakey multipurpose c.
- DeBakey patent ductus c.
- DeBakey peripheral vascular c.
- DeBakey tangential occlusion c.
- ductus c.
- Fogarty Hydrogrip c.
- Glover coarctation c.
- Glover curved c.
- Glover patent ductus c.
- Glover peripheral vascular c.
- Glover vascular c.
- indifferent c.
- Kay aorta c.
- Kelly c.
- Köcher c.
- Lambert-Kay c.
- Lambert-Kay aorta c.
- Mayo c.
- Mixter c.

clamp *(continued)*
mosquito c.
multipurpose c.
multitooth Potts ductus c.
occluding c.
occlusion c.
Ochsner c.
patent ductus c.
Péan c.
peripheral vascular c.
Potts ductus c.
right angle c.
Sarot bronchus c.
Satinsky vascular c.
Schnidt c.
sponge c.
straight mosquito c.
straight vascular c.
tangential occlusion c.
tonsil c.
towel c.
tube-occluding c.
tubing c.
vascular c.
vascular occluding c.
vena cava c.

clamping
cross-c.

claque•ment
c. d'ouverture

Clari•pex

class
heart failure c.

clas•si•fi•ca•tion
Collet and Edwards c. of truncus arteriosus
DeBakey c. of aortic dissection
Heath-Edwards c. of pulmonary vascular disease
Keith-Wagener-Barker c.
Killip's c. of heart disease
New York Heart Association (NYHA) c.

clau•di•cant

clau•di•ca•tion
intermittent c.
jaw c.
venous c.

clau•di•ca•tory

clear•ance
airway c.
drug c.

C-Lex•in

click
late systolic c.
midsystolic c.
ejection c's
systolic c's
systolic ejection c.

click mur•mur syn•drome

Clin•o•ril

clip
ligation c.
wound c.

clo•fi•brate

clo•ni•dine hy•dro•chlo•ride

Clos•trid•i•um
C. perfringens

clos•trid•i•um *pl.* clos•trid•ia

clo•sure
primary c.

clot
agonal c.
agony c.
antemortem c.
blood c.
chicken fat c.
currant jelly c.
distal c.
external c.
heart c.
internal c.
laminated c.
marantic c.

clot *(continued)*
muscle c.
passive c.
plastic c.
postmortem c.
proximal c.
stratified c.
washed c.
white c.

clox•a•cil•lin so•di•um

Clox•a•pen

club•bing
digital c.

clu•pan•o•don•ic acid

cm
centimeter

CMT
circus movement tachycardia

CO
cardiac output

CO_2
carbon dioxide

Co
cobalt

CoA
coenzyme A

co•ag•u•la•tion
c. cascade
common pathway of c.
disseminated intravascular c. (DIC)
extrinsic pathway of c.
c. factors (I–XIIIa)
intrinsic pathway of c.

co•ag•u•lop•a•thy

co•ag•u•lum *pl.* co•ag•u•la

co•arc•ta•tion
c. of aorta
c. of aorta, adult type
c. of aorta, infantile type

co•arc•ta•tion *(continued)*
aortic c.
juxtaductal c.
postductal c.
preductal c.
reversed c.

co•balt

co•caine
c. hydrochloride

Coc•cid•i•oi•des

coc•cid•i•oi•do•my•co•sis

coc•cid•io•my•co•sis

Cock•ayne
C. syndrome

Cock•sackie A vi•rus

Cock•sackie B vi•rus

code
Brownlee pacemaker c.
ICHD pacemaker c.
NASPE specific c.
NBG pacemaker c.
Smyth c.

co•deine
c. phosphate
c. polistirex
c. sulfate

Coe•nen
Henle-C. test

co•en•zyme
c. A
c. Q
c. Q_{10}

coeur
c. en sabot

Cof•fin
C.-Lowry syndrome
C.-Siris syndrome

Co•hen
C. syndrome

coil
Helifix c.
multifilar c.
trifilar c.

COLD
chronic obstructive lung disease

Co•les•tid

co•les•ti•pol
c. hydrochloride

col•ic
biliary c.

co•li•tis
ulcerative c.

col•la•gen
type III c.

col•lapse
cardiovascular c.

col•lar
c. of Stokes

col•lat•er•al
coronary c's

col•lat•er•al•i•za•tion

col•lec•tion
gated list mode c.

Col•let
C. and Edwards classification of truncus arteriosus

col•li•ma•tor
converging c.
diverging c.
high-resolution c.
high-resolution parallel hole c.
high-sensitivity c.
high-sensitivity parallel hole c.
LEAP c.
parallel hole c.
slant hole c.

col•loid

col•o•bo•ma of iris–anal atre•sia syn•drome

col•umn
fleshy c's of heart
plasma exchange c.

co•lum•na *pl.* co•lum•nae
columnae carneae cordis

co•mes *pl.* com•i•tes

com•mis•sion
Intersociety C. for Heart Disease

com•mis•sur•ot•o•my
closed mitral c.
direct vision c.
mitral c.
open c.
open mitral c.

com•pac•tin

com•part•ment
vascular c.

com•pen•sa•tion
broken c.

com•ple•ment

com•plex
anomalous c.
atrial c.
atrial premature c.
Eisenmenger c.
electrocardiographic c.
histocompatibility c.
interpolated premature ventricular c.
Lutembacher's c.
major histocompatibility c. (MHC)
multifocal premature ventricular c's
multiform premature ventricular c's
nodal premature c.

com•plex *(continued)*
pleomorphic premature ventricular c's
polymorphic premature ventricular c's
premature c.
premature atrial c.
premature atrioventricular junctional c.
premature ventricular c.
prothrombinase c.
QRS c.
QS c.
R-on-T premature ventricular c.
transposition c.
ventricular c's
ventricular depolarization c.
ventricular depolarizing c.
ventricular premature c.

com•pli•ance
chamber c.
left ventricular chamber c.
left ventricular diastolic c.
patient c.
pulmonary c.
specific c.
ventricular c.
ventricular diastolic c.

com•po•nent
parallel elastic c.

com•pound
Hurler-Scheie c.

com•pres•sion
chest c.
closed-chest cardiac c.
intermittent pneumatic c.
open-chest cardiac c.

com•pro•mise
airway c.
vascular c.

Comp•ton
C. scattering

con•cen•tra•tion
mean corpuscular hemoglobin c. (MCHC)

con•cre•tio
c. cordis
c. pericardii

con•cus•sion
myocardial c.

con•duc•tion
aberrant c.
aberrant ventricular c.
anomalous c.
anterograde c.
atrioventricular c.
atrioventricular nodal c.
2:1 AV c.
3:2 AV c.
AV nodal c.
c. bundle
cardiac c.
concealed c.
decremental c.
delayed c.
impulse c.
intraventricular c.
retrograde c.
supernormal c.
VA c.
ventricular c.
ventriculoatrial c.

con•duc•tor
hollow core c.
lead c.
Medtronic multifilar c.
multifilar c.
single coil c.
tinsel wire c.
trifilar c.

cone
arterial c.
sarcoplasmic c.

con•fer•ence
Cholesterol Consensus C.
NIH Obesity Consensus C.
Triglyceride Consensus C.

con•ges•tion
active c.
functional c.
hypostatic c.
passive c.
physiologic c.
pulmonary c.
venous c.

Con•ju•gat•ed Es•tro•gens
C.S.D.

con•nec•tion
partial anomalous pulmonary venous c.
pulmonary venous c.
total anomalous pulmonary venous c.
total cavopulmonary c.
univentricular atrioventricular c.

con•nec•tor
Biotronik lead c.
bipolar c.
Cordis c.
Edwards lead c.
General Electric lead c.
lead c.
Medtronic c.
neutral c.
Siemens-Elema lead c.
single pin bipolar c.
unipolar c.

Con•radi
C.-Hünermann syndrome

Con•ray

con•ser•va•tion
blood c.

con•stant
elastic stiffness c.

Con•stant-T

con•stric•tion
arterial c.

con•sump•tion
myocardial oxygen c.

con•sump•tion *(continued)*
oxygen c.

con•tent
mixed venous oxygen c.

con•tour
isoresponse c's

con•tra•cep•tive
oral c.

con•trac•tile

con•trac•til•i•ty
cardiac c.
myocardial c.
ventricular c.

con•trac•tion
atrial premature c.
automatic ventricular c.
cardiac c.
end-diastolic premature ventricular c.
escaped ventricular c.
isometric c.
isotonic c.
isovolumetric c.
isovolumetric left ventricular c.
isovolumic c.
nodal premature c.
premature c.
premature ventricular c.
R-on-T premature ventricular c.
ventricular premature c.

con•trac•tor
Bailey rib c.
rib c.

con•trol
closed loop c. of drug infusion
fuzzy c. of drug infusion

con•tu•sion
cardiac c.
myocardial c.

co•nus *pl.* co•ni
  c. arteriosus

con•vert•ing en•zyme

con•vexo•con•cave

Coo•ley
  C's anemia
  C. atrial retractor
  C. coarctation clamp
  C's disease
  C. multipurpose clamp
  C. patent ductus clamp
  C. pediatric clamp
  C. retractor
  C. vascular clamp
  C. vena cava clamp
  C.-Cutter caged-disk valve

cool•ing
  core c.

COPD
  chronic obstructive pulmonary disease

Cope
  C's needle

cop•per
  c. 62
  c. sulfide

co•pros•ta•nol

cop•ro•ste•rin

co•pros•ter•ol

cor
  c. adiposum
  c. arteriosum
  c. biloculare
  c. bovinum
  c. dextrum
  c. hirsutum
  c. pendulum
  c. pseudotriloculare biatriatum
  c. pulmonale
  c. sinistrum
  c. taurinum

cor *(continued)*
  c. triatriatum
  c. triloculare
  c. triloculare biatriatum
  c. triloculare biventriculare
  c. venosum
  c. villosum

Cor•da•rone

Cor•dis
  C. connector
  C. Omnicor programmer
  C. pulse generator

Cor•gard

Cor•ne•lia de Lange syndrome

cor•o•na•ri•tis

cor•o•nary
  café c.

Cor•o•nary Drug Pro•ject

Cor•o•nary Pri•mary Pre•ven•tion Tri•al

Cor•o•nex

Cor•o•phyl•lin

cor•pus *pl.* cor•po•ra
  corpora arantii
  corpora para-aortica

cor•pus•cle

Cor•ri•gan
  C's disease
  C's pulse
  C's sign

Cor•tef

Cor•ten•e•ma

cor•tex *pl.* cor•ti•ces
  adrenal c.

cor•ti•co•ster•oid

cor•ti•cos•ter•one meth•yl ox•i•dase

cor•ti•cos•ter•one 18-mono•
oxy•gen•ase

cor•ti•co•tro•pin

Cor•ti•foam

cor•ti•sol

Cor•tro•syn

Cor•vi•sart
C's disease

Cor•y•ne•bac•te•ri•um

cos•to•chon•dri•tis

cos•to•ster•nal syn•
drome

co•syn•tro•pin

Co•trim

cough
aneurysmal c.
cardiac c.

cou•lomb

Cou•ma•din

cou•ma•rin

count
blood c.
complete blood c.
erythrocyte c.
leukocyte c.

coun•ter
gamma c.

coun•ter•pul•sa•tion
intra-aortic balloon c.
intra-arterial c.

coun•ter•shock
electrical c.

coup•ling
arterial c.
electromechanical c.
excitation-contraction c.
fixed c.
ventriculoarterial c.

Cour•nand
C. catheter
C. needle

cou•ver•cle

Cox•i•el•la

CPAP
continuous positive airway
pressure

CPB
cardiopulmonary bypass

CPI
carbomethoxyisopropyl
isonitrile

CPK
creatine phosphokinase

CPPT
Coronary Primary
Prevention Trial

CPR
cardiopulmonary
resuscitation

C pro•tein

Cr
chromium

Cra•foord
C. clamp
C. coarctation clamp

Cramp•ton
C's test

cra•nio•syn•os•to•sis–ra•di•
al apla•sia syn•drome

Craw•ford
C. suture ring

crease
ear lobe c.
inguinal skin c.

cre•a•tine ki•nase

cre•a•tine phos•pho•
ki•nase

Creech
C. technique

creep
diaphragmatic c.

cre•na *pl.* cre•nae
c. cordis

crest
infundibuloventricular c.
supraventricular c.
terminal c. of right atrium

Cre•veld
Ellis-van C. syndrome

cri du chat syn•drome

Crile
C. clamp
C. retractor
C.-Wood needle holder

crimp

crimp•er

cri•sis *pl.* cri•ses
hypertensive c.

cris•ta *pl.* cris•tae
c. supraventricularis
c. terminalis atrii dextri

cri•te•ri•on *pl.* cri•te•ria
Dallas criteria
Jones criteria in rheumatic fever diagnosis
Minnesota code criteria

cro•mo•lyn
c. sodium

Cronk•hite
Canada-C. syndrome
C.-Canada syndrome

cross-clamp•ing

cross•match

cross-pro•gram•ming

cross•talk

crown
c. of thorns

CRT
cathode ray tube

cru•or *pl.* cru•o•res

crus *pl.* cru•ra
c. dextrum fasciculi atrioventricularis
c. sinistrum fasciculi atrioventricularis

Cru•veil•hier
C's nodules
C.-Baumgarten murmur

crux *pl.* cru•ces
c. of heart

cryo•ab•la•tion
endocardial c.

cryo•car•dio•ple•gia

cryo•glob•u•lin•emia

cryo•le•sion

cryo•pre•cip•i•tate

cryo•probe

cryo•sur•gery

cryp•to•coc•co•sis

Cryp•to•coc•cus
C. neoformans

cryp•toph•thal•mos syn•drome

crys•tal
piezoelectric c.
sodium iodide scintillation c.

crys•tal•loid

Crys•ti•cil•lin

Crys•to•dig•in

CS
coronary sinus
cycloserine

Cs
cesium

CS (coronary sinus) elec•tro•gram

CT
computed tomography

Cu
copper

Cue•mid

cuff•ing
peribronchial c.

cul•ture
blood c.

cu•pid's bow

cu•ra•re

cu•rie

cur•rent
diastolic c. of energy
diastolic c. of injury
c. of energy
c. of injury
inwardly rectifying c.
K c.
leakage c.
outwardly rectifying c.
pacemaker c.
potassium rectifying c.
systolic c. of energy
systolic c. of injury

curve
cardiac output c.
dye-dilution c.
Frank-Starling c.
hemoglobin-oxygen dissociation c.
indicator-dilution c.
left ventricular pressure-volume c.
length–active tension c.
pressure-natriuresis c.
pressure-volume c.
pulse c.

curve *(continued)*
Starling's c.
thermal dilution c.
thermodilution c.
time-activity c.
venous return c.
ventricular function c.
voltage exponential decay c.

Cush•ing
C's disease
C. forceps
C. pressure response
C's syndrome

cush•ion
intimal c's

cusp
anterior c. of mitral valve
anterior c. of pulmonary valve
anterior c. of tricuspid valve
aortic c.
c's of aortic valve
commissural c's
infundibular c. of tricuspid valve
left c. of aortic valve
left c. of pulmonary valve
marginal c. of tricuspid valve
medial c. of tricuspid valve
posterior c. of aortic valve
posterior c. of mitral valve
posterior c. of tricuspid valve
c's of pulmonary valve
right c. of aortic valve
right c. of pulmonary valve
semilunar c.
semilunar c's of aortic valve
semilunar c's of pulmonary valve
septal c. of tricuspid valve

cus•pis *pl.* cus•pi•des
- c. anterior valvae atrioventricularis dextrae
- c. anterior valvae atrioventricularis sinistrae
- c. anterior valvulae bicuspidalis
- c. anterior valvulae tricuspidalis
- cuspides commissurales
- c. medialis valvulae tricuspidalis
- c. posterior valvae atrioventricularis dextrae
- c. posterior valvae atrioventricularis sinistrae
- c. posterior valvulae bicuspidalis
- c. posterior valvulae tricuspidalis
- c. septalis valvae atrioventricularis dextrae

cut•down
- surgical c.
- venous c.

cu•tis
- c. laxa

Cut•ter
- Cooley-C. caged-disk valve

cut•ter
- wire c.

CV
- cardiovascular

CVD
- cardiovascular disease

CVP
- central venous pressure

CW (continuous wave) Dop•pler imag•ing

c wave

CWI
- cardiac work index

CXR
- chest x-ray

CxR
- chest x-ray

cy•a•no•ac•ryl•ate

cy•a•nose
- c. tardive

cy•a•no•sis
- central c.
- differential c.
- peripheral c.
- c. retinae
- shunt c.
- tardive c.

cy•cle
- cardiac c.
- citric acid c.
- electrical cardiac c.
- forced c.
- Krebs' c.
- mechanical cardiac c.
- restored c.
- returning c.
- tricarboxylic acid c.
- Wenckebach c.

cyc•lic AMP

cyc•lic GMP

cy•clo•oxy•gen•ase

cy•clo•phos•pha•mide

cy•clo•pro•pane

Cy•clo-Pros•tin

cy•clo•spor•ine

cy•clo•thi•a•zide

cyst
- hydatid c.
- pericardial c.
- solitary renal c.

cyst *(continued)*
    springwater c.

cys•ti•cer•co•sis

Cys•to-Con•ray

Cys•to•graf•in

Cys•to•spaz

cy•to•kine

cy•to•meg•a•lo•vi•rus

Cy•to•sar-U

cy•to•sine
    c. arabinoside

cy•to•sta•sis

Cy•tox•an

D

D
atrium and ventricle (pacemaker code)

Da•Costa
D's syndrome

Da•cron
D. patch
D. suture
D. tube graft

DAD
delayed afterdepolarization

Da•la•lone

Dal•mane

damp•ing

dance
brachial d.
hilus d.
St. Vitus' d.

Da•ni•ni
Aschner-D. test

Dan•los
Ehlers-D. syndrome

Dan•tri•um

dan•tro•lene so•di•um

data•bank
Duke Cardiovascular Disease d.

dau•no•my•cin

dau•no•ru•bi•cin
d. hydrochloride

Da•vid•son
D. scapular retractor

Da•vis
D. roller

Day
Riley-D. syndrome

Da•za•mide

daz•ox•i•ben
d. hydrochloride

DBP
diastolic blood pressure

DC
direct current

DCD (differential current density) elec•trode

DCI
digital cardiac imaging

DDAVP
desmopressin acetate

DDD (universal) pace•maker

DDD (universal) pac•ing

DDDR (universal–rate responsive) pace•maker

DDI (atrioventricular sequential) pace•maker

DDI (atrioventricular sequential) pac•ing

deaf•ness

de•ar•te•ri•al•iza•tion

death
brain d.
brainstem d.
sudden d.
sudden cardiac d.
sudden infant d.
voodoo d.

Dea•ver
D. retractor

De•Bakey
D. bulldog clamp

De•Bakey *(continued)*
D. classification of aortic dissection
D. coarctation clamp
D. multipurpose clamp
D. patent ductus clamp
D. peripheral vascular clamp
D. tangential occlusion clamp

Deb•e•trol

deb•ris•o•quin sul•fate

Dec•a•dron

Dec•a•ject

de•can•nu•late

de•can•nu•la•tion

de•cel•er•a•tion

de•cho•les•ter•ol•iza•tion

De•cho•lin

Dec•li•nax

de•com•pen•sa•tion

de•com•po•si•tion
cardiac d.

de•com•pres•sion
cardiac d.
d. of heart
d. of pericardium

de•con•di•tion•ing

de-epi•car•di•al•iza•tion

de•fect
aortic septal d.
aorticopulmonary septal d.
atrial septal d's
atrial ventricular septal d.
atrioseptal d's
atrioventricular canal d.
complete atrioventricular canal d.
doubly committed ventricular septal d.

de•fect *(continued)*
endocardial cushion d's
filling d.
high ventricular septal d.
infracristal ventricular septal d.
muscular ventricular septal d.
noncommitted ventricular septal d.
ostium primum d.
ostium secundum d.
perimembranous ventricular septal d.
primum atrial septal d.
resting thallium d.
secundum atrial septal d.
septal d.
sinus venosus d.
sinus venosus atrial septal d.
subaortic ventricular septal d.
subarterial ventricular septal d.
subpulmonary ventricular septal d.
supracristal ventricular septal d.
ventricular septal d.

de•fer•ox•amine
d. hydrochloride
d. mesylate

de•fib•ril•la•tion

de•fib•ril•la•tor
automatic cardioverter-d.
automatic implantable cardioverter-d.
cardioverter-d.
fully implantable cardioverter-d.
implantable d.
implantable cardioverter-d.
synchronized d.

de•fi•cien•cy
factor XI d.
familial apolipoprotein C-II d.
familial high-density lipoprotein (HDL) d.
familial lipoprotein d.
familial β-lipoprotein d.
familial lipoprotein lipase d.
β-glucuronidase d.
11β-hydroxylase d.
17α-hydroxylase d.
LCAD d.
lecithin:cholesterol acyltransferase (LCAT) d.
lipoprotein lipase (LPL) d.
long chain acyl-CoA dehydrogenase (LCAD) d.
LPL d.
17,20-lyase d.
procoagulant d.
protein-calorie d.

de•fi•cit
pulse d.

de•flec•tion
H d.
His bundle d.
intrinsic d.
intrinsicoid d.
negative d.
positive d.
V d.
voltage d.

de•form•i•ty
buttonhole d.
funnel d.
gooseneck d.
parachute d.
rolled edge d.

de•gen•er•a•tion
angiolithic d.
atheromatous d.
elastoid d.
fibrinoid d.

de•gen•er•a•tion *(continued)*
medial d.
Mönckeberg's d.
myofibrillar d.
myxomatous d.
sclerotic d.

De•hio
D's test

de•hy•dro•cho•les•ter•ol
7-d., activated

de•hy•dro•cho•lic acid

de•hy•dro•em•e•tine

de•hy•dro•gen•ate

de•hy•dro•gen•a•tion

De•jer•ine
Landouzy-D. dystrophy

De•la•di•ol

de Lange
Brachmann-de L. syndrome
de L. syndrome

de•lay
atrioventricular conduction d.
conduction d.
intraventricular conduction d.

Del•bet
D's sign

De•Lee
D.-Hillis obstetric stethoscope

Del•es•tro•gen

de•lir•i•um *pl.* de•lir•ia

Del•ta-Cor•tef

Del•ta•sone

de•mand
myocardial oxygen d.

De•Martel
D. scissors

Dem•er•ol

de Mus•set
de M. sign

den•drite

de•ner•vat•ed

de•ner•va•tion
cardiac d.

den•si•tom•e•try
x-ray d.

den•si•ty
proton d.

de•oxy•cho•late

de•oxy•chol•ic acid

de•oxy•chol•yl•gly•cine

de•oxy•chol•yl•taur•ine

dep•Gyn•o•gen

dep•Med•a•lone

De•po-Es•tra•di•ol

De•po•gen

De•po•ject

de•po•lar•iza•tion
atrial d.
myocardial d.
phase 4 d.
rapid d.
spontaneous d.
ventricular d.

de•po•lar•ize

De•po-Med•rol

De•po•nit

De•po•pred

De•po-Pred•ate

de•pot
fat d.

de•pres•sion
central d.
myocardial d.
precordial ST segment d.
ST segment d.
ventricular d.

Der•ma•lene suture

Der•ma•lon suture

der•ma•ti•tis *pl.* der•ma•tit•i•des
exfoliative d.

der•ma•to•myo•si•tis

Der•o•nil

de•sat•u•ra•tion

de•scent
x d.
y d.

Des•champs
D. needle

des•eth•yl•am•id•a•rone

Des•fer•al

des•fer•ri•ox•amine

de•sip•ra•mine hy•dro•chlo•ride

des•lan•o•side

des•mo•pres•sin
d. acetate

des•mos•ter•ol

Des•y•rel

de•tec•tion
coincidence d.
entry site d.
single photon d.

De•ten•sol

de•ter•mi•na•tion
ejection fraction d.
right heart pressure d.

De•thy•rone

de•vas•cu•lar•iza•tion

De•Vega
D. annuloplasty

de•vi•a•tion
abnormal left axis d.
abnormal right axis d.
axis d.
left axis d.
right axis d.

de•vice
active fixation d.
Adams-DeWeese d.
assist d.
biventricular replacement d.
blood gas exchange d.
cell-washing d.
endocardial fixation d.
external ventricular assist d.
implantable electrical d.
intracaval d.
intracoronary stenting d.
lead fixation d.
left ventricular assist d.
passive fixation d.
pulsatile ventricular assist d.
ventricular assist d.
ventricular assistive d.

De•Weese
Adams-D. device

Dex•a•cen

dex•a•meth•a•sone
d. acefurate
d. acetate
d. dipropionate
d. sodium phosphate

Dex•a•sone

Dex•e•drine

dex•io•car•dia

Dex•on su•ture

Dex•one

dex•ter

dex•trad

dex•tran
d. 40
d. 70
d. 75
high molecular weight d.
low molecular weight d.

dex•tro•car•dia
mirror-image d.
secondary d.

dex•tro•po•si•tion

dex•tro•thy•rox•ine so•di•um

dex•tro-trans•po•si•tion

dex•tro•ver•sion

Dey-Dose Iso•eth•a•rine

Dey-Dose Iso•pro•te•re•nol

Dey-Lute Iso•eth•a•rine

DFP
diastolic filling pressure

DHCA
deep hypothermia circulatory arrest

DHE 45

di•a•be•tes
d. insipidus
d. mellitus (DM)
type II d.

di•ac•e•to•lol

di•a•cyl•glyc•er•ol

di•ag•no•sis
noninvasive d.

di•a•gram
ladder d.
ladder timing d.
pressure-volume d.
vector d.

di•a•gram *(continued)*
Wiggers d.

Di•a•lume

di•al•y•sis
peritoneal d.

Di•a•mox

di•a•phragm
d. transducer

di•as•ta•sis
d. cordis

di•as•to•le
electrical d.

di•a•stol•ic

di•a•ther•my

dia•tri•zo•ate
d. meglumine
d. sodium

Di•az•e•muls

di•az•e•pam

di•az•ox•ide

Di•ben•zy•line

DIC
disseminated intravascular coagulation

di•clox•a•cil•lin so•di•um

di•crot•ic

di•cro•tism

di•cu•ma•rol

Die•ker
Miller-D. syndrome

di•et
low cholesterol d.
low fat d.
low salt d.
low sodium d.
salt-free d.
salt-restricted d.
sodium-restricted d.

Dieth•rich
D. coronary artery set
D. coronary scissors
D. valve scissors

di•eth•yl•stil•bes•trol
d. diphosphate
d. dipropionate

dif•fer•ence
arteriovenous oxygen d.

di•gam•ma•car•boxy•glu•tam•ic acid

Di•George
D. sequence
D's syndrome

dig•i•tal•is
d. glycosides

dig•i•tal•iza•tion

dig•i•tox•in

di•glyc•er•ide

di•gox•in

di•hy•dro•cho•les•ter•ol

di•hy•dro•er•got•amine mes•y•late

Di•hy•dro•er•got•amine-San•doz

Di•lan•tin

dil•a•ta•tion
balloon d.
bootstrap d.
d. of the heart
idiopathic d.
post-stenotic d.
ventricular d.

di•la•tion
balloon d.
reactive d.

di•la•tor
aortic d.
Garrett d.
Gerbode valve d.

di•la•tor *(continued)*
mitral valve d.
myocardial d.
Tubbs mitral valve d.
Tubbs valve d.

Di•la•trate

dil•ti•a•zem hy•dro•chlo•ride

di•mar•gar•in

di•men•sion
jet d.
ventricular d.

Di•o•val

di•pha•sic

di•phen•hy•dra•mine
d. citrate
d. hydrochloride

Di•phen•yl•an

di•phen•yl•hy•dan•to•in
d. sodium

di•phos•pha•ti•dyl•glyc•er•ol

2,3-di•phos•pho•glyc•er•ate

diph•the•ria

dip•lo•car•dia

di•pole

Di•prid•a•cot

di•py•rid•a•mole

Dirck
D's fibrils

dis•a•bil•i•ty
cardiovascular d.

disc
see *disk*

dis•charge
accelerated automatic d.
self-d.
systolic d.

dis•ease (see also under *syndrome*)

dis•ease *(continued)*
accelerated coronary artery d.
accelerated graft vascular d.
Addison's d.
Albright's d.
amyloid heart d.
Anderson-Fabry d.
aortic thromboembolism d.
arteriosclerotic d.
atherosclerotic d.
atherosclerotic coronary artery d.
Beau's d.
Becker's d.
beriberi heart d.
biliary d.
Bouveret's d.
broad-beta d.
broncho-obstructive d.
Buerger's d.
carcinoid heart d.
carcinoid valve d.
carotid arterial d.
cerebrovascular d.
Charcot-Marie-Tooth d.
cholesteryl ester storage d. (CESD)
chronic obstructive lung d.
chronic obstructive pulmonary d. (COPD)
congenital heart d. (CHD)
congestive heart d. (CHD)
Cooley's d.
coronary artery d. (CAD)
coronary heart d. (CHD)
Corrigan's d.
Corvisart's d.
Cushing's d.
Döhle d.
Duroziez's d.
Ebstein's d.
Emery-Dreifuss d.
endomyocardial d.
end-stage renal d.
eosinophilic endomyocardial d.

dis•ease *(continued)*
Fabry's d.
Fallot's d.
fibroplastic d.
fixed obstructive
coronary d.
floating-beta d.
Friedländer's d.
Gaisböck's d.
Gaucher's d.
glycogen storage d.
Goldstein's d.
heart d.
Heberden's d.
Heller-Döhle d.
hepatic d.
Hodgkin's d.
Hodgson's d.
Horton's d.
Huchard's d.
Hutchinson-Gilford d.
hypertensive pulmonary
vascular d.
iron storage d.
ischemic heart d.
Johnson-Stevens d.
Kawasaki d.
kidney d.
Klemperer's d.
Kussmaul's d.
Kussmaul-Maier d.
Laënnec's d.
Landouzy's d.
legionnaires' d.
Lenègre's d.
Lev's d.
Libman-Sacks d.
Little's d.
Löffler's d.
Lobstein's d.
Lutembacher's d.
Lyme d.
McArdle's d.
Mondor's d.
Monge's d.
Morquio's d.
Moschcowitz's d.
multivalvular d.

dis•ease *(continued)*
multivessel coronary
artery d.
myocardial d.
neoplastic d.
nonischemic heart d.
obstructive lung d.
Opitz's d.
Osler's d.
Osler-Weber-Rendu d.
Paget d.
parathyroid d.
pericardial d.
pericardial restrictive d.
peripheral arterial d.
peripheral vascular d.
polycystic kidney d.
Pompe's d.
premature coronary
artery d.
primary electrical d.
pulmonary collagen
vascular d.
pulmonary parenchymal d.
pulmonary vascular
obstructive d.
pulmonary veno-
occlusive d.
pulmonic valve d.
pulseless d.
Raynaud's d.
Reiter's d.
renal d.
renal artery d.
renal parenchymal d.
Rendu-Osler-Weber d.
restrictive pericardial d.
rheumatic heart d.
rheumatic mitral valve d.
rheumatic valvular
heart d.
Roger's d.
Rougnon-Heberden d.
Roussy-Lévy d.
Schönlein's d.
Schönlein-Henoch d.
sickle-cell d.
single vessel d.

dis•ease *(continued)*
Steinert's d.
Still's d.
Stokes-Adams d.
syphilitic heart d.
Takayasu's d.
Takayasu-Ohnishi d.
Tangier d.
temperate endomyocardial d.
Thomsen's d.
three vessel d.
thromboembolic d.
thyrocardiac d.
thyroid d.
thyrotoxic heart d.
Tietze's d.
traumatic heart d.
tricuspid valve d.
tropical endomyocardial d.
valvular heart d.
von Recklinghausen's d.
von Willebrand's d.
Weil's d.
Werlhof's d.
Whipple's d.
Willebrand's d.
Winiwarter-Buerger d.

disk
intercalated d.
intervertebral d's
Pyrolyte d.

di•so•pyr•amide
d. phosphate

dis•or•der
acute cerebral d.
atrial septal d.
LDL-receptor d.
pericardial d.
septal d.

dis•play
cine d.
endless loop d.

Dispos-a-Med Iso•eth•a•rine

Dispos-a-Med Iso•pro•te•re•nol

dis•sec•tion
aortic d.
blunt d.
finger d.
pseudoaortic d.
sharp d.

dis•sec•tor
sponge d.

dis•so•ci•a•tion
atrial d.
atrioventricular d.
auriculoventricular d.
AV d.
electromechanical d.
interference d.
d. by interference
isorhythmic atrioventricular d.

dis•ten•si•bil•i•ty

dis•ten•tion
jugular venous d.

dis•tress
respiratory d.

dis•tur•bance
conduction d.

Di•u•car•din

Diu•chlor H

Di•u•lo

di•ure•sis *pl.* di•ure•ses
osmotic d.

di•uret•ic
K^+-sparing d.
loop d.
osmotic d.
potassium-sparing d's

Di•uril

di•ver•tic•u•lum *pl.* di•ver•tic•u•la
aortic d.

di•ver•tic•u•lum *(continued)*
  Heister's d.

Dix•ar•it

diz•zi•ness

do•bu•ta•mine
  d. hydrochloride
  d. tartrate

Do•bu•trex

do•co•sa•hexa•eno•ic acid

Dodge
  Sheehan and D. method

Döhle
  D. disease
  D.-Heller aortitis
  Heller-D. disease

dom•per•i•done

do•nee

do•nor

DOO (atrioventicular asynchronous sequential) pace•maker

DOO (dual chamber asynchronous) pace•maker

do•pa
  L-d.

Do•pa•met

do•pa•mine
  d. hydrochloride

do•pa•mine be•ta-hy•drox•y•lase

Do•par

dop•ex•amine
  d. hydrochloride

Dop•pler
  color D.
  color D. echocardiography
  color D. imaging
  color flow D.

Dop•pler *(continued)*
  color flow D. echocardiography
  color flow D. imaging
  color flow imaging D. echocardiography
  continuous wave D. echocardiography
  continuous wave D. ultrasonography
  CW (continuous wave) D.
  directional D.
  D. color flow imaging
  D. color flow mapping
  D. echocardiography
  D. imaging
  D. mapping
  D. recording
  D. signal
  D. study
  D. ultrasonography
  D. ultrasound
  laser D. velocimetry
  pulse D.
  pulsed D. echocardiography
  pulsed wave D. echocardiography
  pulsed wave D. ultrasonography
  PW (pulsed wave) D.
  real time D.

Dor•en•dorf
  D's sign

Dor•i•glute

dor•sad

dor•sal

dor•so•in•ter•cos•tal

dor•so•lat•er•al

dor•so•me•di•an

dor•so•me•si•al

dor•so•ven•trad

DORV
double-outlet right ventricle

dose
absorbed d.
systemic d.

Dot•ter
D. technique

Doug•las
D. bag method

Down
D. syndrome

dox•a•zo•sin
d. mesylate

dox•e•pin hy•dro•chlo•ride

doxo•ru•bi•cin
d. hydrochloride

Do•yen
D. rib raspatory

DPTI
diastolic pressure–time index

Drag•er
Shy-D. syndrome

drain
current d.

drain•age
gravity d.
isolated partial anomalous pulmonary venous d.

Drei•fuss
Emery-D. disease
Emery-D. muscular dystrophy

dress•ing
pressure d.

Dres•sler
D's syndrome

DRG
diagnosis-related group

drift
rate d.

drive
ventilatory d.

dri•ver
Utah pneumatic heart d.

dromo•graph

drom•o•trop•ic

dro•per•i•dol

drop•sy
cardiac d.

Drum•mond
D's sign

DTI
diastolic time interval

DTPA
diethylenetriaminepenta-acetic acid

D-tu•bo•cu•ra•rine

Du•chenne
D. muscular dystrophy
D's sign
D's type

duct
collecting d.
d's of Cuvier
medullary collecting d.

duc•tus *pl.* duc•tus
patent d. arteriosus
reversed d. arteriosus

dull

dull•ness
Gerhardt's d.
tympanitic d.

Du•o•trate

dupp

Du•ra•cil•lin

Du•ra-Es•trin

Du•ra•gen

Du•ra•lith

Du•ra•lone

Du•ra•morph

Du•ra•pam

Du•ra•phyl

du•ra•tion
pulse d.

Du•ret•ic

Du•ri•cef

Du•ro•med•ics
D. bileaflet valve
D. prosthesis

Du•ro•zi•ez
D's disease
D's murmur
D's sign

Dutch•er
D. lead

Du•val
D. lung forceps

Du•void

DVI (atrioventricular sequential) pace•maker

DVI (atrioventricular sequential) pac•ing

dwarf•ism
Robinow d.

Dy•cil

dye
indocyanine green d.
radiopaque d.

dy•nam•ics
membrane lipid d.
microvascular d.

dy•namo•scope

dy•na•mos•co•py

Dy•na•pen

Dy•no•thel

Dy•ren•i•um

dys•ar•te•ri•ot•o•ny

dys•au•to•no•mia
familial d.

dys•be•ta•lipo•pro•tein•emia
familial d.

dys•cra•sia
blood d.

dys•en•ce•pha•lia splanch•no•cys•ti•ca

dys•fi•brin•o•gen•emia

dys•func•tion
left ventricular d.
mitral valve d.
papillary muscle d.
platelet d.
segmental left ventricular d.
sinus node d.
systolic left ventricular d.
ventricular d.

dys•gen•e•sis
gonadal d.

dys•ki•ne•sia
d. intermittens

dys•ki•ne•sis
systolic d.

dys•ki•net•ic

dys•lipo•pro•tein•emia
primary d.
secondary d.

dys•lipo•pro•tein•emic

dys•or•ia

dys•or•ic

dys•os•to•sis
mandibulofacial d.

dys•pla•sia
- arrhythmogenic right ventricular d.
- arteriohepatic d.
- camptomelic d.
- chondroectodermal d.
- fibromuscular d.
- fibrous d.
- geleophysic d.
- oculoauricular vertebral d.
- right ventricular d.
- thanatophoric d.

dysp•nea
- cardiac d.
- exertional d.
- expiratory d.
- inspiratory d.
- nocturnal d.
- paroxysmal nocturnal d.
- pulmonary d.

dys•rhyth•mia
- perioperative d.
- sinus d.
- supraventricular d.

dys•syn•chro•ny

dys•ta•sia
- Roussy-Lévy hereditary areflexic d.

dys•tro•phy
- Becker's d.
- Becker's muscular d.
- Duchenne type muscular d.
- Emery-Dreifuss muscular d.
- Erb's d.
- facioscapulohumeral muscular d.
- Landouzy d.
- Landouzy-Dejerine d.
- limb-girdle muscular d.
- muscular d.

E

η
absolute viscosity

EAD
early afterdepolarization

E-Base

Eberth
E's line

EBF
effective pulmonary blood flow

Eb•stein
E's anomaly
E's disease
E's sign

E-CABG
endarterectomy and coronary artery bypass grafting

ECC
Emergency Cardiac Care
extracorporeal circulation

ECG
electrocardiogram

Echi•no•coc•cus

echi•no•coc•cus *pl.* echi•no•coc•ci

echo
amphoric e.
metallic e.
ventricular e.

echo•car•dio•gram (see also under *echocardiography*)
T-M e.
time-motion (T-M) e.

echo•car•di•og•ra•phy
A-mode e.
B-mode e.
color Doppler e.

echo•car•di•og•ra•phy *(continued)*
color flow Doppler e.
color flow imaging Doppler e.
color flow two-dimensional e.
continuous wave Doppler e.
contrast e.
cross-sectional e.
CW (continuous wave) Doppler e.
deductive e.
deductive two-dimensional e.
epicardial e.
exercise e.
fetal e.
imaging e.
invasive e.
M-mode e.
pulsed Doppler e.
pulsed wave Doppler e.
real time two-dimensional e.
PW (pulsed wave) Doppler e.
transesophageal e.
transthoracic e.
two-dimensional e.

echo•ge•ni•ci•ty

echo•pho•no•car•di•og•ra•phy

ECHO vi•rus

echo•vi•rus

EC/IC (extracranial/intracranial) by•pass

eclamp•sia

ECMO
extracorporeal membrane oxygenation

ec•ta•sia
- annuloaortic e.
- e. of aorta
- coronary artery e.
- diffuse arterial e.
- hypostatic e.

ec•top•ic

ec•to•py
- ventricular e.

E-Cyp•i•o•nate

ED
- end diastole

Edec•rin

ede•ma
- alveolar e.
- angioneurotic e.
- brawny e.
- cardiac e.
- cardiogenic pulmonary e.
- cerebral e.
- dependent e.
- high-altitude pulmonary e.
- idiopathic cyclic e.
- interstitial e.
- interstitial pulmonary e.
- myocardial e.
- neurogenic pulmonary e.
- noncardiogenic pulmonary e.
- pitting e.
- pulmonary e.

ed•e•tate
- e. calcium disodium
- e. disodium
- e. sodium
- e. trisodium

EDRF
- endothelium-derived relaxing factor

ed•ro•pho•ni•um
- e. chloride

EDTA
- ethylenediaminetetra-acetic acid

EDV
- end-diastolic volume

Ed•wards
- Carpentier-E. valve
- Collet and E. classification of truncus arteriosus
- E. lead connector
- Heath-E. classification of pulmonary vascular disease
- Starr-E. caged-ball valve
- Starr-E. prosthetic valve

EERP
- extended endocardial resection procedure

E.E.S.

EEV
- encircling endocardial ventriculotomy

EF
- ejection fraction

ef•fect
- Anrep e.
- Bainbridge e.
- fetal alcohol e's
- fetal hydantoin e's
- fetal rubella e's
- fetal trimethadione e's
- fetal valproate e's
- fetal warfarin e's
- Frank-Starling e.
- inotropic e.
- jet e.
- negative inotropic e.
- positive inotropic e.
- proarrhythmic e.
- snowplow e.
- Venturi e.

ef•fu•sion
- pericardial e.

Eg•gle•ston
  Bradbury-E. syndrome
  E's method

Eh•lers
  E.-Danlos syndrome

ei•co•sa•no•ate

ei•co•sa•no•ic acid

ei•co•sa•noid

ei•co•sa•pen•ta•eno•ic acid (EPA)

Ei•ken•el•la
  E. corrodens

Ein•tho•ven
  E's formula
  E's galvanometer
  E's law
  E's triangle

Ei•sen•men•ger
  E. complex
  E's syndrome
  tetralogy of E.

ejec•tion
  rapid e.
  reduced e.
  e. shell

EKG
  electrocardiogram

elas•tic•i•ty
  volume e.

elas•tom•e•ter

elas•tom•e•try

El•a•vil

elec•tro•aug•men•ta•tion

elec•tro•car•dio•gram
  bipolar e.
  esophageal e.
  intracardiac e.
  scalar e.
  unipolar e.

elec•tro•car•di•o•graph

elec•tro•car•di•og•ra•phy
  ambulatory e.
  esophageal e.
  exercise e.
  intrabronchial e.
  intracardiac e.
  intracavitary e.
  12-lead e.
  long term e.
  precordial e.
  resting e.
  signal averaged e.

elec•tro•car•dio•ver•sion

elec•tro•cau•ter•iza•tion

elec•tro•cau•tery

elec•tro•chem•i•cal

elec•trode
  anode e.
  ball e.
  ball-tip e.
  barb e.
  bipolar e.
  button e.
  cathode e.
  DCD e.
  differential current density e.
  dish e.
  electronic pacemaker wire e.
  endocardial e.
  endocardial pacing e.
  endocardial permanent e.
  epicardial e.
  epicardial pacing e.
  epicardial permanent e.
  epimyocardial e.
  esophageal e.
  esophageal pill e.
  exploring e.
  fixation e.
  ground e.
  hand-held e.
  Helifix e.

elec•trode *(continued)*
indifferent e.
Laserpor e.
low polarization threshold e.
low voltage threshold e.
monopolar e.
needle e.
pacemaker e.
pacing e.
e. paddle
permanent e.
pill e.
platinum e.
platinum-iridium e.
porous e.
porous surface e.
porous tipped e.
reference e.
ring e.
screw-in e.
solid e.
solid tip e.
spring-loaded barb e.
surface e.
target tip e.
temporary e.
temporary pacemaker e.
titanium e.
totally porous e.
transseptal e.
transvenous e.
transvenous permanent e.
unipolar e.
vitreous carbon e.

elec•tro•gen•ic

elec•tro•gram
atrial e.
bipolar e.
bipolar atrial e.
bipolar His e.
coronary e.
coronary sinus e.
CS e.
esophageal e.
high right atrial e.
His e.

elec•tro•gram *(continued)*
His bundle e.
intra-atrial e.
intracardiac e.
low right atrial e.
right ventricular e.
right ventricular apical e.
sinus node e.
unipolar e.
ventricular e.

elec•tro•graph

elec•trog•ra•phy

elec•tro•im•mu•no•as•say

elec•tro•ky•mo•gram

elec•tro•ky•mo•graph

elec•tro•ky•mog•ra•phy

elec•tro•lyte

elec•tro•me•chan•i•cal

elec•tron

elec•tro•pho•re•sis

elec•tro•phys•i•ol•o•gy
cardiac e.
clinical cardiac e.

elec•tro•sur•gery

elec•tro•ver•sion

elec•tro•vert

El•e•ma
Siemens-E. lead connector
Siemens-E. pacemaker lead
Siemens-E. ribbon lead

el•e•ment
automatic e.
conductile e.
contractile e.
series elastic e.

el•e•va•tion
ST segment e.

el•e•va•tor
  Freer e.
  nasal e.
  neurosurgical e.
  Penfield e.
  periosteum e.

El•gi•loy
  E. alloy
  E. strut

ELISA
  enzyme-linked immunosorbent assay

Elix•i•con

Elix•o•min

Elix•o•phyl•lin

Elle•stad
  E. protocol

El•lis
  E.-van Creveld syndrome

Els•ner
  E's asthma

em•bo•lec•to•my
  femoral e.
  pulmonary e.
  transvenous pulmonary e.

em•bo•li

em•bol•ic

em•bol•i•form

em•bo•lism
  air e.
  aortic e.
  arterial e.
  atheromatous e.
  bacillary e.
  bland e.
  bone marrow e.
  capillary e.
  coronary e.
  crossed e.
  direct e.
  fat e.

em•bo•lism *(continued)*
  infective e.
  massive pulmonary e.
  miliary e.
  multiple e.
  nonparadoxical e.
  nonthrombotic pulmonary e.
  oil e.
  pantaloon e.
  paradoxical e.
  plasmodium e.
  pulmonary e.
  recurrent pulmonary e.
  saddle e.
  spinal e.
  submassive pulmonary e.
  thrombotic pulmonary e.
  trichinous e.
  venous e.

em•bo•li•za•tion
  paradoxical e.
  poppet e.
  septic e.

em•bo•lo•my•cot•ic

em•bo•lus *pl.* em•bo•li
  air e.
  cancer e.
  cellular e.
  cerebral e.
  fat e.
  foam e.
  obturating e.
  pulmonary e.
  riding e.
  saddle e.
  straddling e.
  tumor e.

em•bouche•ment
  paradoxical e.

em•bry•op•a•thy
  retinoic acid e.
  warfarin e.

emer•gen•cy
  hypertensive e.

Em•ery
  E.-Dreifuss disease
  E.-Dreifuss muscular dystrophy

em•e•tine
  e. hydrochloride

Em•i•trip

em•phy•se•ma
  subcutaneous e.

em•py•e•ma
  e. of pericardium

E-My•cin

enal•a•pril
  e. maleate

en•cain•ide
  e. hydrochloride

en•cap•su•la•tion
  hermetic e.

en•car•di•tis

en•ceph•a•lop•a•thy
  hypertensive e.
  metabolic e.

end•an•gi•itis

end•an•gi•um

end•aor•tic

end•aor•ti•tis
  bacterial e.

end•ar•ter•ec•to•my
  carotid e.
  gas e.
  transaortic e.

end•ar•te•ri•al

end•ar•ter•itis

end•ar•te•ri•um

end•ar•ter•op•a•thy
  digital e.

end-ar•tery

En•dep

end-di•as•tol•ic

en•do•an•eu•rys•mor•rha•phy

en•do•an•gi•itis

en•do•aor•ti•tis

en•do•ar•ter•itis

en•do•car•di•al

en•do•car•di•op•a•thy

en•do•car•dit•ic

en•do•car•di•tis
  abacterial thrombotic e.
  acute e.
  atypical verrucous e.
  bacterial e.
  e. benigna
  e. chordalis
  chronic e.
  constrictive e.
  Coxsackie e.
  culture-negative e.
  fetal e.
  fungal e.
  gonococcal e.
  infectious e.
  infective e.
  e. lenta
  Libman-Sacks e.
  Löffler's e.
  Löffler's fibroplastic e.
  Löffler's parietal fibroplastic e.
  malignant e.
  marantic e.
  mural e.
  mycotic e.
  nonbacterial thrombotic e.
  nonbacterial verrucous e.
  noninfective e.
  nonvalvular infective e.
  parietal e.
  e. parietalis fibroplastica
  prosthetic valve e.
  pulmonic e.
  rheumatic e.

en•do•car•di•tis *(continued)*
rickettsial e.
right-side e.
septic e.
staphylococcal e.
streptococcal e.
subacute bacterial e.
syphilitic e.
tuberculous e.
ulcerative e.
valvular e.
vegetative e.
verrucous e.
viridans e.

en•do•car•di•um

en•do•cy•to•sis
receptor-mediated e.

en•do•myo•car•di•al

en•do•myo•car•di•tis

en•do•my•si•al

en•do•nu•cle•ase
restriction e.

en•do•peri•car•di•al

en•do•peri•car•di•tis

en•do•peri•myo•car•di•tis
reverse e.

en•do•phle•bi•tis
proliferative e.

en•dor•phin

en•dos•co•py

en•do•stetho•scope

en•do•the•li•al

en•do•the•lin

en•do•the•li•um *pl.* en•do•the•lia

en•do•tho•rac•ic

en•do•tox•in

en•do•vas•cu•li•tis

en•do•ve•ni•tis

en•do•ve•nous

en•dox•in

end point
therapeutic e.

en•dra•la•zine
e. mesylate

end-sys•tol•ic

En•dur-Ac•in

En•du•ron

en•e•ma *pl.* en•e•mas, e•nem•a•ta
barium e.
sodium polystyrene sulfonate e.

en•er•gom•e•ter

en•er•gy
current of e.
diastolic current of e.
systolic current of e.

en•flu•rane

En•kaid

en•large•ment
cardiac e.
e. of heart
left atrial e.
right atrial e.

En•lon

En•o•vil

enox•i•mone

en•train

en•train•ment

en•zyme
angiotensin-converting e.
cardiac e's
converting e.
lysosomal e.
myocardial e.

EOL
    end of (battery) life

eo•sin•o•phil

eo•sin•o•phil•ia

E-Pam

Ephed

ephed•rine
    e. hydrochloride
    e. sulfate

epi•car•di•al

epi•car•di•ec•to•my

epi•car•di•um

epi•du•ral

Epi•morph

epi•neph•rine
    e. bitartrate

Epi•Pen Au•to•In•jec•tor

ep•i•stax•is

Ep•i•tol

E point

ep•o•pro•sten•ol

epoxy

EPS
    electrophysiologic study

EPSS
    E point–septal separation

Ep•stein
    E.-Barr virus

ep•ta•sta•tin

equa•tion
    Gorlin e.
    Fick e.
    Nernst e.
    Poiseuille e. (Hagenbach extension)
    Starling e.

equi•lib•ri•um
    multigated e.

equiv•a•lent
    anginal e.

Erb
    E's dystrophy

Erd•heim
    E's cystic medial necrosis

er•gom•e•ter
    bicycle e.

er•gom•e•try
    bicycle e.

er•go•no•vine
    e. maleate

er•got
    e. alkaloids

Er•go•trate

eri•tri•tyl
    e. tetranitrate

ERP
    endocardial resection procedure

eru•cic acid

Eryc

Ery•Ped

Er•y•sip•elo•thrix

Ery-Tab

er•y•the•ma
    e. marginatum
    e. multiforme

eryth•ri•tyl
    e. tetranitrate

Eryth•ro

Eryth•ro•cin

Eryth•ro•cot

eryth•ro•cy•to•sis

eryth•ro•gen•in

Eryth•ro•mid

eryth•ro•my•cin
e. acistrate
e. estolate
e. ethylcarbonate
e. ethylsuccinate
e. gluceptate
e. glucoheptonate
e. lactobionate
e. propionate
e. propionate lauryl sulfate
e. stearate
e. stinoprate

eryth•ro•phe•re•sis

Eryth•ro•zone

ES
end systole

es•cape
nodal e.
vagal e.
ventricular e.

Esch•e•rich•ia
E. coli

Es•i•drix

Es•ka•lith

Es•march
E's tourniquet

es•mo•lol
e. hydrochloride

esoph•a•ge•al

esoph•a•gi•tis

ESR
erythrocyte sedimentation rate

EST
exercise stress test

es•ter
cholesteryl e.

Es•ti•nyl

Es•trace

Es•tra-D

Es•tra•derm

Es•tra-L

Es•tra•tab

Es•tra•val

Es•tro-Cyp

Es•tro•fem

es•tro•gen
conjugated e's
esterified e's

Es•tro•ject

Es•tro•nol

Es•tro•vis

ESV
end-systolic volume

ESVI
end-systolic volume index

eth•a•cryn•ic acid

etham•bu•tol hy•dro•chlo•ride

eth•a•nol

ether
diethyl e.

Eth•i•bond suture

Eth•i•flex suture

Eth•i•lon suture

eth•mo•car•di•tis

Eth•mo•zine

Eth•rane

Eth•ril

eth•y•lene•di•a•mine•tet•ra-a•ce•tic acid

Eti•bi

etom•i•date

eto•po•side

eu•an•gi•ot•ic

eu•die•mor•rhy•sis

Eu•ler
    E. number

Eu•li•pos

eu•rhyth•mia

Eu•ro•pe•an Cor•o•nary Sur•gery Stu•dy

eu•sys•to•le

eu•sys•tol•ic

eu•thy•roid sick syn•drome

eval•u•a•tion
    left ventricular diastolic function e.
    ventricular function e.

Ewart
    E's sign

ex•change
    gas e.
    pulmonary gas e.
    sodium-potassium e.

ex•ci•ta•bil•i•ty

ex•ci•ta•tion
    anomalous atrioventricular e.
    reentrant e.
    supernormal e.

ex•ci•to•vas•cu•lar

ex•cres•cence
    Lambl's e's

ex•er•cise
    active e.
    cardiovascular e.
    continuous e.
    dynamic e.
    intermittent e.
    isometric e.
    isometric handgrip e.

ex•er•cise *(continued)*
    isotonic e.
    passive e.
    static e.
    subjective maximal e.
    submaximal e.
    supine e.
    upright e.

ex•er•tion
    rating of perceived e.

ex•it block
    high threshold e.b.
    sinoatrial e.b.
    sinus e.b.
    Wenckebach e.b.

Ex•na

exo•car•di•al

ex•om•pha•los-ma•cro•glos•sia-gi•gan•tism syn•drome

ex•oph•thal•mos

ex•pan•sion
    infarct e.

ex•per•i•ment
    Müller's e.
    Valsalva's e.

ex•pi•ra•tion

ex•ten•der
    artificial plasma e.

ex•tra-an•a•tom•ic

ex•tra•car•di•al

ex•tra•cor•po•re•al

ex•tra•peri•car•di•al

ex•tra•stim•u•lus

ex•tra•sys•to•le
    atrial e.
    atrioventricular e.
    auricular e.
    auriculoventricular e.
    concealed ventricular e.
    infranodal e.

ex·tra·sys·to·le *(continued)*
  interpolated e.
  nodal e.
  retrograde e.
  return e.
  ventricular e.

ex·tra·tho·rac·ic

ex·tra·vas·cu·lar

ex·tra·ven·tric·u·lar

eye

F

F
fluorine

Fa•bry
Anderson-F. disease
F's disease
F's syndrome

FACC
Fellow of the American College of Cardiology

fa•ci•es *pl.* fa•ci•es
f. anterior cordis
f. dextra cordis
f. diaphragmatica cordis
f. inferior cordis
f. lateralis cordis
mitral f.
mitrotricuspid f.
f. pulmonalis cordis
f. sternocostalis cordis

fac•tor
angiogenesis f.
antihemophilic f.
atrial natriuretic f. (ANF)
autocrine f.
coagulation f's (I–XIII)
cryoprecipitated antihemophiliac f.
endothelial-derived relaxant f.
endothelium-derived relaxing f.
epidermal growth f.
fibroblast growth f.
growth f.
Hageman f. (HF)
myocardial depressant f. (MDF)
paracrine f.
platelet f's (1–4)
platelet-derived growth f.
psychosocial f.
rheumatoid f. (RF)

fac•tor *(continued)*
tissue f.
transforming growth f. alpha
transforming growth f. beta
tumor necrosis f. (TNF)
f. V
von Willebrand's f.
Willebrand's blood coagulation f.
f. X
f. XI

FAI
functional aerobic impairment

fail•ure
acute circulatory f.
acute heart f.
backward heart f.
cardiac f.
chronic heart f.
circulatory f.
congestive heart f. (CHF)
contrast-induced acute renal f.
diastolic heart f.
end-stage chronic renal f.
forward heart f.
heart f.
high-output heart f.
intractable heart f.
left-sided heart f.
left ventricular f.
low-output heart f.
myocardial f.
phasic pacemaker f.
pulmonary f.
refractory heart f.
renal f.
right-sided heart f.
right ventricular f.
systolic heart f.

faint•ing
  hysterical f.

faint•ness

Fal•lot
  F's disease
  F's syndrome
  F's tetrad
  pentalogy of F.
  tetralogy of F.
  trilogy of F.

falx *pl.* fal•ces
  f. septi

Fan•co•ni
  F's anemia
  F's pancytopenia
  F's pancytopenia syndrome

Far•ber
  F's lipogranulomatosis

FAS
  fetal alcohol syndrome

fas•cia *pl.* fas•ciae
  f. adherens
  endothoracic f.
  f. endothoracica

fas•ci•cle

fas•cic•u•lo•ven•tric•u•lar

fas•cic•u•lus *pl.* fas•cic•cu•li
  f. atrioventricularis

fat
  body f.
  dietary f.
  epicardial f.
  monounsaturated f.
  neutral f.
  polyunsaturated f.
  saturated f.
  unsaturated f.

fa•tigue
  hemodynamic f.

fat•ty

fat•ty ac•id
  essential f.a.
  free f.a's (FFA)
  monounsaturated f.a's
  n-3 f.a's
  nonesterified f.a's (NEFA)
  ω-3 f.a's
  ω-6 f.a's
  omega-3 f.a's
  omega-6 f.a's
  polyunsaturated f.a's
  saturated f.a's
  unsaturated f.a's

5-FC
  flucytosine

F-de•oxy•glu•cose

FDG
  F-deoxyglucose
  2-fluoro-2-deoxyglucose

Fe
  iron

feed•back
  PID (proportional plus integral plus derivative) f.

feed•through

Feil
  Klippel-F. sequence

felt
  Teflon f.

Fem•i•none

Fem•o•gen

Fem•o•gex

fem•o•ral

fem•o•ro•fem•o•ral

fen•es•tra•tion
  aorticopulmonary f.
  aortopulmonary f.

fen•ta•nyl cit•rate

Fen•ton
F. reaction

Fer•gie
F. needle

Fer•gu•son
F. needle

fer•ro•mag•net•ic

fe•tal al•co•hol syn•drome

fe•tal face syn•drome

fe•tal hy•dan•to•in syn•drome

fe•tal ru•bel•la syn•drome

fe•tal tri•meth•a•di•one syn•drome

fe•tal war•fa•rin syn•drome

fe•ver
Q f.
relapsing f.
Rocky Mountain spotted f.
yellow f.

FFP
fresh frozen plasma

FG syn•drome

fi•ber
accelerating f's
accelerator f's
afferent f's
augmentor f's
bulbospiral f's
cardiac accelerator f's
cardiac depressor f's
cardiac pressor f's
conducting f's
depressor f's
dietary f.
efferent f's
fasciculoventricular f's
forklike f's
Henle's f's
impulse-conducting f's

fi•ber *(continued)*
insoluble f.
James f.
Mahaim f's
motor f.
myocardial f's
nodoventricular f's
pressor f's
Purkinje f's
sensory f.
sinospiral f's
soluble f.
terminal conducting f's of Purkinje

fibril
Dirck's f's

fi•bril•la•tion
atrial f.
auricular f.
cold f.
flutter-f.
postoperative atrial f.
ventricular f.

fi•brin

fi•brin•o•gen

fi•brin•oid

fi•bri•nol•y•sis

fi•bri•no•lyt•ic

fi•bri•no•pep•tide A

fi•bro•elas•to•ma

fi•bro•elas•to•sis
endocardial f.

fi•bro•ma
cardiac f.

fi•bro•nec•tin

fi•bro•plas•tic

fi•bro•sar•co•ma
cardiac f.

fi•bro•sis
African endomyocardial f.
biventricular endomyocardial f.
cystic f.
endomyocardial f.
fetal endomyocardial f.
left ventricular endomyocardial f.
progressive interstitial pulmonary f.
right ventricular endomyocardial f.
tropical endomyocardial f.
venous f.

Fick
continuous F. method
direct F. method
direct F. procedure
direct F. technique
F. equation
F. formula
F. method
F. oxygen method
F. principle
F. procedure
F. technique
rebreathing F. method

Fied•ler
F's myocarditis

field
f. of view

fig•ure
hexaxial f.
triaxial f.

fill•ing
diastolic f.
early diastolic f.
rapid ventricular f.
reduced ventricular f.
ventricular f.

film
anteroposterior f.
AP f.

film *(continued)*
cine f.
plain f.
serial AP f.

fil•ter
bandpass f.
Kimray-Greenfield f.
Mobin-Uddin f.
umbrella f.

fil•ter•ing
arrhythmia f.

fil•tra•tion
arterial line f.

Fink
Autenrieth and F's method

Fi•no•chiet•to
F. retractor

first and sec•ond bran•chi•al arch syn•drome

Fisch•er
F's sign

fis•sure
Henle's f's

fis•tu•la *pl.* fis•tu•lae, fis•tu•las
aortocaval f.
aortoenteric f.
aortopulmonary f.
arteriovenous f.
coronary arteriovenous f.
coronary artery f.
pulmonary arteriovenous f.
pulmonary arteriovenous f., congenital
renal f.
traumatic f.

Flack
F's node
F's test
Keith-F. node

Flag•yl

FLASH (fast low-angle shot) tech•nique

flat•ness

flat•ten•ing
  T wave f.

Flax•e•dil

fle•cai•nide
  f. acetate

Flex•on steel su•ture

Flint
  F's murmur

flop•py valve syn•drome

flow
  arterial blood f.
  blood f.
  circulatory f.
  collateral f.
  coronary f.
  coronary blood f.
  effective blood f.
  microcirculatory blood f.
  myocardial blood f.
  pulmonary f.
  pulmonary blood f.
  pulsatile f.
  residual f.
  shunt f.
  systemic f.
  systemic blood f.

flow•me•ter
  blood f.
  electromagnetic f.

flow tract

Flu•clox

flu•clox•a•cil•lin

flu•cy•to•sine

flu•de•oxy•glu•cose F 18

flu•id
  crystalloid f.
  pericardial f.
  pleural f.

flu•o•res•ce•in

flu•o•rine
  f. 18

5-flu•o•ro•cy•to•sine

^{18}F 2-flu•o•ro-2-de•oxy•glu•cose

flu•o•ro•roent•ge•nog•ra•phy

flu•o•ro•scope

flu•o•ro•scop•ic

flu•o•ros•co•py
  cardiac digital f.

5-flu•o•ro•ura•cil

Flu•o•sol

Flu•o•sol-DA

Flu•o•thane

flu•ox•e•tine
  f. hydrochloride

flu•raz•e•pam hy•dro•chlo•ride

flut•ter
  atrial f.
  auricular f.
  impure f.
  pure f.
  ventricular f.

flut•ter-fi•bril•la•tion

fo•cal

fo•cus *pl.* fo•ci
  ectopic f.
  ventricular f.

Fo•gar•ty
  F. balloon catheter
  F. catheter

Fo•gar•ty *(continued)*
F. Hydrogrip clamp

fold
Marshall's f.
Rindfleisch's f's
vestigial f. of Marshall

Fo•lex

fol•ic acid

Fon•tan
F's operation
F. procedure
F. repair

fo•ra•men *pl.* fo•ra•mi•na
aortic f.
Galen's f.
oval f. of fetus
f. ovale
f. ovale cordis
patent f. ovale
foramina of smallest veins of heart
thebesian foramina
foramina thebesii
f. venae cavae
vena caval f.
foramina venarum minimarum atrii dextri
foramina venarum minimarum cordis
Vieussen's foramina

For•ane

force
extravascular compressive f.
peak twitch f.
reserve f.
rest f.
Starling f's

for•ceps
Adson f.
Cushing f.
DeBakey tissue f.
Duval lung f.

for•ceps *(continued)*
hemostatic f.
lung f.
Martin f.
Rumel thoracic f.
Russian f.
Russian tissue f.
Singley f.
smooth f.
smooth tissue f.
sponge f.
thoracic f.
thumb f.
tissue f.
toothed f.
vascular tissue f.

for•ma•lin

for•mu•la *pl.* for•mu•lae, for•mu•las
Bazett's f.
bullet f.
Einthoven's f.
Fick f.
Hamilton-Stewart f.
Simpson's rule f.

fos•sa *pl.* fos•sae
antecubital f.
oval f. of heart
f. ovalis cordis
subclavicular f.

Foy•gen

frac•tion
ejection f.
exercise ejection f.
first third filling f.
global ejection f.
left ventricular ejection f.
regurgitant f.
right ventricular ejection f.

frag•ment
Fab f.

frag•men•ta•tion
f. of myocardium

Fram•ing•ham Heart Stu•dy

Fran•ce•schet•ti
F.-Klein syndrome
Treacher Collins-F. syndrome

Frank
F. electrode system
F's law
F. lead system
F. XYZ leads
F.-Starling curve
F.-Starling effect
F.-Starling law
F.-Starling mechanism of the heart
F.-Starling phenomenon
F.-Starling principle
F.-Starling relation

Frän•kel
F's treatment

Fra•ser
F. syndrome

Fra•zier
F. suction tip

Freer
F. elevator

frem•i•tus
friction f.
pericardial f.

French
F. catheter
F. eye needle
F. scale
F. unit
F.-Robinson catheter

fre•quen•cy
Nyquist f.
resonant f.

fri•a•ble

Fri•as
Opitz-F. syndrome

fric•tion
f. rub

Frie•dreich
F's ataxia
F's sign
F's syndrome

frole•ment

Frosst•image Al•bu•min

Frosst•image DTPA

Frosst•image MAA

Frosst•image Sul•fur Col•loid

fruc•tose bis•phos•phate al•do•lase

fruc•tose 1,6-di•phos•phate al•do•lase

5-FU
fluorouracil

fuch•sin•o•phil•ia

Fu•ci•din

ful•gu•ra•tion

Ful•vi•cin

func•tion
cardiac f.
diastolic f.
left ventricular f.
right ventricular f.
ventricular f.
ventricular diastolic f.

fun•dus *pl.* fun•di

fun•gal

Fun•gi•zone

fun•gus *pl.* fun•gi

fu•nic•u•lus *pl.* fu•nic•u•li
hepatic f.

fu•nis
  f. brachii

F (French) unit

fun•nel
  mitral f.

fu•ro•sem•ide

Fur•o•side

fur•row
  atrioventricular f.

fu•si•dic acid

F waves

G

G
    ventricular gradient (electrocardiography)

Ga
    gallium

Gab•bay
    Meadox-G. unicusp pericardial valve

Gad
    G's hypothesis

gad•o•lin•i•um

Gais•böck
    G's disease
    G's syndrome

Ga•len
    G's foramen

gal•la•mine tri•eth•io•dide

gal•li•um
    g. 68

gal•lop
    atrial g.
    diastolic g.
    fourth heart sound g.
    fourth sound gallop g.
    mid-diastolic g.
    presystolic g.
    protodiastolic g.
    S_3 g.
    S_4 g.
    summation g.
    third heart sound g.
    third sound g.
    ventricular g.

gal•va•nom•e•ter
    Einthoven's g.
    string g.
    thread g.

gam•ma•car•boxy•glu•tam•ic acid

gan•gli•on *pl.* gan•glia, gan•gli•ons
    Bezold's g.
    Bidder's ganglia
    cardiac ganglia
    ganglia cardiaca
    Ludwig's g.
    Remak's g.
    sinoatrial g.
    sinus g.
    ventricular g.
    Wrisberg's g.

gan•gli•on•ic

gan•grene
    angiosclerotic g.
    embolic g.
    static g.
    symmetric g.
    thrombotic g.
    venous g.

Gan•ong
    Lown-G.-Levine syndrome

Gan•ta•nol

Gan•tri•sin

gan•try

Ganz
    Swan-G. catheter
    Swan-G. monitoring catheter

gap
    auscultatory g.
    excitable g.
    silent g.

Ga•ra•my•cin

gar•ment
    pneumatic antishock g.

Gar•rett
    G. dilator

Gärt•ner
G's phenomenon
G's tonometer

gas
aortic blood g.
blood g.

Gas•kell
G's bridge

Gas•tro•crom

Gas•tro•graf•in

gate
d g.
F g.
h g.
m g.

gate•post
chordal g.

gat•ing
ECG g.
electrocardiographic g.
in-memory g.
physiological g.
prospective g.
retrospective g.

Gau•cher
G's disease

gauge
Brown and Sharp (B&S) g.
USP g.

gauze
Surgicel g.

Ga•vis•con

Gd
gadolinium

gel
aluminum hydroxide g.
EKG electrode g.
ultrasound transmission g.

Gel•foam

Gel•pi
G. retractor

gem•fib•ro•zil

Ge•na•bid

Gen•er•al Elec•tric lead connector

gen•er•a•tor
bipolar impulse g.
dual-chamber impulse g.
electronic pulse g.
implantable pulse g.
impulse g.
multiprogrammable impulse g.
nuclear-powered impulse g.
pulse g.
R wave–inhibited pulse g.
synchronous pulse g.

gen•in

Gen•si•ni
G. coronary arteriography catheter

Gen•ta•cin

gen•ta•mi•cin
g. sulfate

Ge•o•pen

Ger•bode
G. valve dilator

Ger•dy
G's interarticular loop

Ger•hardt
G's dullness
G's triangle

Ger•i•mal

Ger•old
Baller-G. syndrome

GEX
graded exercise test

GGT
γ-glutamyltransferase

GGTP
γ-glutamyl transpeptidase

Gib·bon
G.-Landis test

Gib·son
G. murmur
G's vestibule

Gied·i·on
Langer-G. syndrome
Schinzel-G. syndrome

Giertz
Stille-G. rib shears

gi·gan·tism
atrial g.

Gil·ford
Hutchinson-G. disease
Hutchinson-G. syndrome

giv·ing-up–giv·en-up re·sponse

gland
adrenal g.
arterial g.
carotid g.
intercarotid g.
parathyroid g's
pituitary g.
thyroid g.
Zuckerkandl's g.

Glas·gow
G's sign

Glenn
G. operation
G. procedure
G. shunt

glob·u·lin
antilymphocyte g. (ALG)
antithymocyte g. (ATG)

glo·mec·to·my

glo·mer·u·lo·ne·phri·tis
acute g.
chronic g.

glo·mic

glo·moid

glo·mus *pl.* glo·me·ra
glomera aortica
g. caroticum
carotid g.
jugular g.
g. jugulare

Glov·er
G. coarctation clamp
G. curved clamp
G. patent ductus clamp
G. peripheral vascular clamp
G. vascular clamp

glu·ca·gon

Gluck
G. rib shears

glu·co·cor·ti·coid

glu·co·cor·ti·co·ster·oid
adrenal g.

glu·cose
g.-insulin-potassium

glu·cose-6-phos·phate de·hy·dro·gen·ase (G6PD)

glu·cose-6-phos·phate isom·er·ase

glue
cryoprecipitate-thrombin calcium fibrin g.
cyanoacrylate g.
topical fibrin g.

glu·tam·ic-ox·alo·ace·tic trans·am·i·nase (GOT)

glu·tam·ic-ox·alo·ace·tic trans·fer·ase

glu•tam•ic-py•ru•vic trans•am•i•nase (GPT)

γ-glu•ta•myl•trans•fer•ase (GGT)

γ-glu•ta•myl trans•pep•ti•dase

glu•ta•ral•de•hyde

glu•teth•i•mide

glyc•er•ide

glyc•er•in

glyc•er•ol

glyc•er•yl
g. trinitrate
g. trioleate
g. tripalmitate

gly•co•che•no•de•oxy•cho•late

gly•co•che•no•de•oxy•cho•lic acid

gly•co•cho•late

gly•co•cho•lic acid

gly•co•gen stor•age dis•ease

gly•co•lip•id

gly•col•y•sis
aerobic g.
anaerobic g.

gly•co•pyr•ro•late

gly•co•side
cardiac g.
digitalis g's

Gly•rol

gm
gram

GMP
guanosine monophosphate

G-My•cin

goi•ter

goi•ter *(continued)*
retrosternal g.

gold
g.-195m

Gold•blatt
G. kidney

Gol•den•har
G's syndrome

Gold•schei•der
G's percussion

Gold•stein
G's disease

Goltz
G. syndrome
Gorlin-G. syndrome

Good•ale
G.-Lubin catheter

Gore-Tex
G. shunt
G. surgical membrane

Gor•lin
G. equation
G. syndrome
G.-Goltz syndrome

GOT
glutamic-oxaloacetic transaminase

Gott
G. shunt

Gou•let
G. retractor

gout

Gow•ers
G. sign

GPD
glucose phosphate dehydrogenase

G6PD
glucose-6-phosphate dehydrogenase

GPT
glutamic-pyruvic transaminase

gra•di•ent
aortic pressure g.
electrochemical g.
left ventricular outflow g.
mitral g.
systolic g.
transvalvular pressure g.
ventricular g.

grad•ing
hemodynamic g.

graft
allogeneic g.
aortic g.
arterial g.
artificial g.
autogenous g.
bifurcated g.
bifurcated vessel g.
bovine g.
coronary artery bypass g. (CABG)
Dacron tube g.
Dacron vessel g.
heterologous g.
heteroplastic g.
homologous g.
homoplastic g.
isogeneic g.
isologous g.
isoplastic g.
knitted g.
mammary artery g.
natural Y sequential vein g.
patch g.
prosthetic g.
prosthetic patch g.
prosthetic tube g.
saphenous vein g.
straight g.

graft *(continued)*
straight tube g.
straight vessel g.
syngeneic g.
tube g.
vascular g.
vein g.
woven g.
woven prosthetic tube g.

graft•ing
coronary bypass g.

Gra•ham Steell
G.S's murmur

gran•ule
atrial g's
specific atrial g's

gran•u•lo•cy•to•pe•nia

gran•u•lo•ma•to•sis
allergic g.
lymphomatoid g.
Wegener's g.

graph•ite

GRASS (gradient recalled acquisition in a steady state) tech•nique

grav•i•do•car•di•ac

Great•bach
Chardack-G. pacemaker

green
indocyanine g.

Green•field
Kimray-G. filter

Gri•ful•vin

Gris•ac•tin

gris•eo•ful•vin

Gri•so•vin

Groc•co
Orsi-G. method

groove
- atrioventricular g.
- auriculoventricular g.
- deltopectoral g.
- interatrial g.
- interventricular g., anterior
- interventricular g. of heart
- interventricular g., inferior
- interventricular g., posterior

ground

group
- diagnosis-related g's

Gru•ber
- G's syndrome
- Meckel-G. syndrome

Gruen•tzig
- G. balloon catheter
- G. technique

G syn•drome

guan•a•benz
- g. acetate
- g. sulfate

guan•a•drel sul•fate

guan•eth•i•dine
- g. monosulfate
- g. sulfate

guan•fa•cine
- g. hydrochloride

guan•o•sine
- g. diphosphate (GDP)
- g. monophosphate (GMP)
- g. triphosphate (GTP)

Guer•rei•ro
- Machado-G. test

guid•ance
- fluoroscopic g.

guide•wire
- J-tipped g.
- steel g.
- steerable g.

Guil•lain
- G.-Barré syndrome

Gunn
- G's crossing sign
- G's sign

GXT
- graded exercise test

gyne•co•mas•tia

Gyn•o•gen

H

H
    bundle of His
    hydrogen

h
    hecto-
    hour

Ha•ber
    H.-Weiss reaction

Hae•mon•et•ics Cell Saver

Hae•moph•i•lus
    H. aphrophilus
    H. influenzae
    H. paraphrophilus

haem•or•rha•gia

Hag•e•man
    H. factor

Ha•gen•bach
    H. extension of Poiseuille equation

Haight
    H. rib raspatory

Hal•ci•on

Hal•dol

Hale
    H's piesimeter

half-life
    biological h.-l.
    elimination h.-l.
    physical h.-l.

Half•prin

Hall
    H's sign
    Medtronic-H. prosthetic valve
    Medtronic-H. tilting-disk valve
    Pallister-H. syndrome

Hal•ler
    H's tripod

Hal•lion
    H's test

hal•o•peri•dol
    h. decanoate

hal•o•thane

ham•ar•to•ma
    cardiac h.

Ham•il•ton
    H.-Stewart formula

Ham•man
    H's murmur
    H's sign
    H.-Rich syndrome

Hamp•ton
    H's hump

Han•cock
    H. bioprosthetic valve
    H. porcine prosthetic valve
    H. porcine xenograft

hand•grip
    isometric h.

Han•lon
    Blalock-H. atrial septectomy
    Blalock-H. operation

HAPE
    high-altitude pulmonary edema

hard•ness
    water h.

Har•ring•ton
    H. retractor

Hartz•ler
    H. LPS catheter

Hay
    H.-Wells syndrome

HBD
    hydroxybutyrate dehydrogenase

H de•flec•tion

HDFP
    Hypertension Detection and Follow-up Program

HDL
    high-density lipoprotein

HDL_1

HDL_2

HDL_3

He
    helium

Hea•ney
    H. needle holder

heart
    abdominal h.
    addisonian h.
    air-driven artificial h.
    amyloid h.
    armored h.
    armour h.
    artificial h.
    athlete's h.
    athletic h.
    atrophic h.
    beer h.
    beriberi h.
    boat-shaped h.
    bony h.
    booster h.
    bovine h.
    cervical h.
    chaotic h.
    drop h.
    dynamite h.
    electrohydraulic h.
    encased h.
    extracorporeal h.
    fat h.

heart *(continued)*
    fatty h.
    fetal h.
    fibroid h.
    flask-shaped h.
    frosted h.
    hairy h.
    hanging h.
    horizontal h.
    hypertensive h.
    hyperthyroid h.
    hypoplastic h.
    hypoplastic left h.
    icing h.
    intracorporeal h.
    Jarvik 7 artificial h.
    left h.
    mechanical h.
    myxedema h.
    nonfailing h.
    ox h.
    paracorporeal h.
    parchment h.
    pear-shaped h.
    pectoral h.
    pendulous h.
    pulmonary h.
    Quain's fatty h.
    rheumatic h.
    right h.
    round h.
    sabot h.
    semihorizontal h.
    semivertical h.
    stone h.
    stony h.
    suspended h.
    systemic h.
    tabby cat h.
    three-chambered h.
    thrush breast h.
    tiger h.
    tiger lily h.
    thyrotoxic h.
    tobacco h.
    total artificial h.
    Traube's h.
    triatrial h.

heart *(continued)*
- trilocular h.
- univentricular h.
- Utah artificial h.
- vertical h.
- wandering h.
- water-bottle h.
- wooden-shoe h.

heart block
- atrioventricular h.b.
- AV h.b.
- bifascicular h.b.
- bundle-branch h.b.
- complete h.b.
- congenital h.b.
- congenital complete h.b.
- divisional h.b.
- familial h.b.
- fascicular h.b.
- first degree h.b.
- incomplete h.b.
- interventricular h.b.
- intra-atrial h.b.
- intraventricular h.b.
- Mobitz h.b.
- Mobitz second degree h.b.
- Mobitz type I second degree h.b.
- Mobitz type II second degree h.b.
- partial h.b.
- periinfarction h.b.
- SA h.b.
- second degree h.b.
- sinoatrial h.b.
- third degree h.b.
- Wenckebach h.b.

heart dis•ease
- beriberi h.d.
- congenital h.d.
- ischemic h.d.
- nonischemic h.d.
- rheumatic h.d.
- syphilitic h.d.
- thyrotoxic h.d.
- traumatic h.d.
- valvular h.d.

heart driv•er
- Utah pneumatic h.d.

heart fail•ure
- acute h.f.
- acute congestive h.f.
- backward h.f.
- chronic h.f.
- congestive h.f.
- diastolic h.f.
- forward h.f.
- high output h.f.
- intractable h.f.
- left-sided h.f.
- left ventricular h.f.
- low output h.f.
- refractory h.f.
- right-sided h.f.
- right ventricular h.f.
- systolic h.f.

heart mur•mur
- apical mid-diastolic h.m.
- apical systolic h.m.
- atrioventricular flow rumbling h.m.
- Austin Flint h.m.
- continuous h.m.
- diastolic h.m.
- ductus h.m.
- early systolic h.m.
- ejection h.m.
- functional h.m.
- Graham Steell h.m.
- holosystolic h.m.
- late systolic h.m.
- mid-diastolic h.m.
- midsystolic h.m.
- systolic h.m.
- ventricular filling h.m.

heart sound
- first h.s.
- fourth h.s.
- second h.s.
- single second h.s.
- third h.s.

Heath
H.-Edwards classification of pulmonary vascular disease

heave
parasternal h.

Heb•er•den
H's asthma
H's disease
Rougnon-H. disease

Heim
H.-Kreysig sign

Heim•lich
H. maneuver

Heis•ter
H's diverticulum

he•li•um

he•lix

Hel•ler
Döhle-H. aortitis
H.-Döhle disease

hem•ado•ste•no•sis

hema•dy•na•mom•e•try

hem•an•gi•ec•ta•sia

hem•an•gi•ec•ta•sis

hem•an•gio•en•do•the•li•o•ma

hem•an•gi•o•ma

hem•an•gio•peri•cyte

hem•an•gio•sar•co•ma

he•ma•to•crit

hem•a•to•ma *pl.* hem•a•tomas
aneurysmal h.
dissecting h.

hem•a•to•ma•nom•e•ter

hem•a•to•peri•car•di•um

hem•a•tor•rhea

hemi•block
left anterior h.
left posterior h.

hemi•car•dia
h. dextra
h. sinistra

hemi•sphyg•mia

he•mo•chro•ma•to•sis
idiopathic h.

he•mo•clip

he•mo•di•al•y•sis

he•mo•dy•nam•ic

he•mo•dy•nam•ics

he•mo•dy•na•mom•e•try

he•mo•glo•bin
mean corpuscular h.
stroma-free h.

he•mol•y•sis
chronic intravascular h.

he•mo•ma•nom•e•ter

he•mo•peri•car•di•um

he•mo•phil•ia
vascular h.

he•mo•pi•ezom•e•ter

he•mo•pneu•mo•me•di•as•ti•num
subclavian h.

he•mo•pneu•mo•peri•car•di•um

he•mop•ty•sis
cardiac h.

he•mor•rhage
arterial h.
brain h.
essential h.
exsanguinating h.
h. per rhexin
reperfusion-induced h.
splinter h's

he•mor•rhage *(continued)*
subungual h.
venous h.

he•mor•rha•gen•ic

he•mor•rha•gic

he•mor•rhag•ip•a•rous

he•mor•rhea

he•mo•sid•er•o•sis
pulmonary h.
transfusional h.

he•mo•stat
Kelly h.
Mayo h.
mosquito h.
straight h.

he•mo•stat•ic

he•mo•tho•rax

HeNe (helium-neon) la•ser

Hen•le
H's elastic membrane
H's fenestrated membrane
H's fibers
H's fissures
H.-Coenen test

He•noch
H's purpura
H.-Schönlein purpura
H.-Schönlein syndrome
Schönlein-H. purpura
Schönlein-H. syndrome

Hep•a•lean

hep•a•rin
h. calcium
low molecular weight h.
h. sodium

hep•ar•i•nized

Hep•a•rin Leo

he•pat•ic tri•glyc•er•ide lip•ase

hep•a•ti•tis *pl.* hep•a•ti•ti•des
viral h.

hep•a•to•gram

hep•a•tog•ra•phy

hep•a•to•meg•a•ly

hep•a•to•sple•no•meg•a•ly

hep•ta•de•ca•no•ic acid

hep•ta•no•ate

hep•ta•no•ic acid

Her•ing
Traube-H. waves

her•nia
hiatal h.

her•o•in

Hes•pan

Hess
H. capillary test

het•a•starch

het•ero•clad•ic

het•ero•di•ag•no•sis

het•ero•graft
porcine h.

het•er•ol•o•gous

het•er•ol•o•gy

het•ero•phy•i•a•sis

het•ero•pla•sia

het•ero•plas•tic

het•ero•plas•tid

het•ero•plas•ty

het•ero•tax•ia

het•ero•trans•plant

het•ero•trans•plan•ta•tion

hexa•dec•a•no•ate

hexa•dec•a•no•ic acid

Hex•a•drol

hexa•no•ate

hex•a•no•ic acid

HF
  Hageman factor (coagulation Factor XII)

Hg
  mercury

hi•a•tus
  aortic h.
  h. aorticus
  vena caval h.

hi•ber•na•tion
  myocardial h.

Hill
  H's sign

Hil•lis
  DeLee-H. obstetric stethoscope

Hines
  H. and Brown test

His
  bundle of H.
  H. band
  H. bundle deflection
  H. bundle electrogram
  H. electrogram
  H. spindle
  H.-ventricular (H–V) interval
  H.-Purkinje conduction time
  H.-Purkinje system
  Kent-H. bundle

his•ta•mine

his•tan•ox•ia

His•tan•til

his•tio•cyte
  cardiac h.

his•to•com•pa•ti•bil•i•ty

his•to•com•pat•i•ble

his•to•in•com•pat•i•bil•i•ty

his•to•in•com•pat•i•ble

His•to•plas•ma

his•to•plas•mo•sis

HIV
  human immunodeficiency virus

HLA
  histocompatibility locus A
  histocompatibility locus antigen
  human leukocyte antigen
  human lymphocyte antigen
  hypoplastic left atrium

HMG CoA (hy•droxy•meth•yl•glu•ta•ryl CoA) re•duc•tase

Hodg•kin
  H's disease
  H.-Huxley model

Hodg•son
  H's disease

hold•er
  needle h.
  prosthetic valve h.
  wire needle h.

hol•i•day heart syn•drome

Hol•len•horst
  H. plaques

holo•di•a•stol•ic

holo•sys•tol•ic

Holt
  H.-Oram syndrome

Hol•ter
  H. monitor
  H. monitoring

Holz•knecht
H's space

Ho•man
H's sign

ho•meo•sta•sis
potassium h.

ho•mo•clad•ic

ho•mo•cys•tin•uria

ho•mo•graft

ho•mol•o•gous

ho•mol•o•gy

ho•mo•plas•tic

ho•mo•plas•ty

ho•mo•trans•plant

Hon•o•lu•lu Heart Pro•gram

Hon•vol

hook
nerve h.

Hope
H's sign

Hor•mo•gen De•pot

hor•mone
adrenocorticotropic h.
antidiuretic h.
female h's
gonadal h's
growth h. (GH)
ketogenic h's
lipolytic h's
natriuretic h.
parathyroid h.
steroid h's
thyroid h's
vasopressor h.

Hor•ner
H's syndrome

Hor•ton
H's arteritis
H's disease

Hor•ton *(continued)*
H's syndrome

HPO
high-pressure oxygenation

HR
heart rate

HRA (high right atrial) elec•tro•gram

HRCT
high-resolution computed tomography

H re•gion

Hu•chard
H's disease

Hughes
H.-Stovin syndrome

hum
cervical venous h.
venous h.

hu•mor•al

hump
Hampton's h.

Hü•ner•mann
Conradi-H. syndrome

Hun•ter
H. detachable balloon occluder
H's operation
H's syndrome
H.-Hurler syndrome

Hur•ler
Hunter-H. syndrome
H. cell
H's syndrome
H.-Scheie compound
H.-Scheie compound syndrome

Hutch•in•son
H.-Gilford disease
H.-Gilford syndrome

Hux•ley
    Hodgkin-H. model

H–V (His-ventricular) in•ter•val

H wave

hy•da•tism

Hy•der•gine

hy•dra•la•zine
    h. hydrochloride
    h. polistirex

hy•dra•zine

Hy•drex

hy•dro•car•bon
    halogenated h.

hy•dro•car•dia

Hy•dro-chlor

hy•dro•chlo•ro•thi•a•zide

hy•dro•cho•les•ter•ol

hy•dro•cor•ti•sone
    h. aceponate
    h. acetate
    h. butyrate
    h. cyclopentylpropionate
    h. cypionate
    h. hemisuccinate
    h. sodium phosphate
    h. sodium succinate
    h. valerate

Hy•dro•cor•tone

hy•dro•cy•an•ic acid

Hy•dro-D

Hy•dro•DI•U•RIL

hy•dro•flu•me•thi•a•zide

hy•dro•gen
    h. peroxide

hy•dro•gen•ate

hy•dro•gen•a•tion

Hy•dro•mox

hy•dro•ne•phro•sis

hy•dro•peri•car•di•tis

hy•dro•peri•car•di•um

hy•dro•pneu•mo•peri•car•di•um

hy•drops
    h. pericardii

hy•dro•sphyg•mo•graph

hy•dro•tho•rax

hy•droxy•am•phet•amine hy•dro•bro•mide

3-hy•droxy•bu•ty•rate de•hy•dro•gen•ase

β-hy•droxy•bu•ty•rate de•hy•dro•gen•ase

hy•droxy•cho•les•ter•ol

hy•droxy•eth•yl starch

hy•drox•yl

11β-hy•drox•y•lase

17α-hy•drox•y•lase

18-hy•drox•y•lase

21-hy•drox•y•lase

hy•droxy•meth•yl•glu•ta•ryl-CoA re•duc•tase

hy•droxy•meth•yl•glu•ta•ryl-CoA re•duc•tase (NADPH)

17α-hy•droxy•pro•ges•ter•one al•do•lase

3β-hy•droxy-Δ^5-ste•roid de•hy•dro•gen•ase

hy•droxy•urea

Hy•gro•ton

Hy•lo•rel

hyo·scine
  h. hydrobromide

hyo·scy·amine
  h. hydrobromide

Hy·paque

Hy·paque-Cys·to

Hy·paque Me·glu·mine

Hy·paque So·di·um

hy·per·acute

hy·per·al·do·ster·on·ism

hy·per·al·pha·lipo·pro·tein·emia

hy·per·be·ta·lipo·pro·tein·emia

hy·per·cal·ce·mia
  idiopathic infantile h.

hy·per·cal·ci·ne·mia

hy·per·cap·nia

hy·per·cho·les·ter·emia

hy·per·cho·les·ter·emic

hy·per·cho·les·ter·in·emia

hy·per·cho·les·ter·ol·emia
  essential h.
  familial h.
  polygenic h.
  primary h.

hy·per·cho·les·ter·ol·emic

hy·per·cho·les·ter·ol·ia

hy·per·chy·lo·mi·cron·emia

hy·per·co·ag·u·la·ble

hy·per·con·trac·til·i·ty

hy·per·di·crot·ic

hy·per·di·cro·tism

hy·per·dy·nam·ic

hy·per·emia
  collateral h.
  passive h.
  reactive h.
  venous h.

hy·per·emic

hy·per·eo·sin·o·phil·ic

hy·per·es·tro·gen·emia

hy·per·gam·ma·glob·u·lin·emia

hy·per·glob·u·lin·emia
  polyclonal h.

hy·per·gly·ce·mia

hy·per·ka·le·mia

hy·per·ki·ne·mia

hy·per·ki·ne·sis

hy·per·ki·net·ic heart syn·drome

hy·per·li·pe·mia
  carbohydrate-induced h.
  combined fat- and carbohydrate-induced h.
  endogenous h.
  essential familial h.
  exogenous h.
  fat-induced h., familial
  mixed h.

hy·per·lip·id·emia
  combined h.
  familial h., type V
  familial combined h.
  mixed h.
  multiple lipoprotein–type h.
  remnant h.

hy·per·lipo·pro·tein·emia
  acquired h.
  familial h.
  Lp(a) h.

hy·per·mag·ne·se·mia

hy•per•na•tre•mia

hy•per•ne•phro•ma

hy•per•os•mo•lar•i•ty

hy•per•para•thy•roid•ism
- primary h.
- secondary h.

hy•per•pla•sia
- adrenal h.
- congenital adrenal h.
- lipoid h.

hy•per•po•lar•iza•tion

hy•per•pre•be•ta•lipo•pro•tein•emia
- familial h.

hy•per•res•o•nance

hy•per•sen•si•tive

hy•per•sen•si•tive ca•rot•id si•nus syn•drome

hy•per•sen•si•tiv•i•ty
- cardioinhibitory carotid sinus h.
- carotid sinus h.
- vagal carotid sinus h.
- vasodepressor carotid sinus h.

hy•per•sphyx•ia

Hy•per•stat

hy•per•telo•rism-hy•po•spa•di•as syn•drome

hy•per•ten•sion
- accelerated h.
- accelerated-malignant h.
- arterial h.
- borderline h.
- chronic h.
- diastolic h.
- drug-induced h.
- episodic h.
- essential h.
- gestational h.
- Goldblatt h.

hy•per•ten•sion *(continued)*
- idiopathic h.
- labile h.
- left atrial h.
- low-renin h.
- low-renin essential h.
- low risk h.
- malignant h.
- maternal h.
- mild h.
- neurogenic h.
- pale h.
- paroxysmal h.
- pediatric h.
- portal h.
- pregnancy-induced h.
- primary h.
- primary pulmonary h.
- pulmonary h.
- red h.
- renal h.
- renal vascular h.
- renovascular h.
- secondary h.
- secondary pulmonary h.
- symptomatic h.
- systemic h.
- systemic venous h.
- systolic h.
- transient h.
- vascular h.
- venous h.
- volume-dependent h.

Hy•per•ten•sion De•tec•tion and Fol•low-up Stu•dy

hy•per•ten•sive

hy•per•ten•sor

hy•per•ther•mia
- malignant h.

hy•per•ther•mic

hy•per•thy•roid•ism
- amiodarone-induced h.
- apathetic h.

hy•per•tri•glyc•er•i•de•mia
familial h.
sporadic h.

hy•per•tro•phy
asymmetrical septal h.
biventricular h.
cardiac h.
cardiac concentric h.
concentric left ventricular h.
left ventricular h.
lipomatous h. of the interatrial septum
myocardial h.
right ventricular h.
ventricular h.
volume load h.

hy•per•uri•ce•mia

hy•per•vas•cu•lar

hy•per•ven•ti•la•tion

hy•per•vi•ta•min•o•sis
h. D

hyp•not•ic

hy•po•al•bu•min•emia

hy•po•al•do•ster•on•ism
hyporeninemic h.

hy•po•be•ta•lipo•pro•tein•emia
familial h.

hy•po•cal•ce•mia

hy•po•cal•ce•mic

hy•po•cho•les•te•re•mia

hy•po•cho•les•te•re•mic

hy•po•cho•les•ter•in•emia

hy•po•cho•les•ter•ol•emia

hy•po•cho•les•ter•ol•emic

hy•po•chon•dri•a•sis

hy•po•dy•na•mia
h. cordis

hy•po•dy•nam•ic

hy•po•func•tion

hy•po•gly•ce•mia

hy•po•ka•le•mia

hy•po•ki•ne•mia

hy•po•ki•ne•sia

hy•po•ki•ne•sis

hy•po•ki•net•ic

hy•po•li•pe•mia

hy•po•lip•id•emic

hy•po•lipo•pro•tein•emia

hy•po•mag•ne•se•mia

hy•po•mag•ne•se•mic

hy•po•me•lia-hy•po•tri•cho•sis-fa•cial hem•an•gi•o•ma syn•drome

hy•po•na•tre•mia
hyperlipemic h.

hy•po•para•thy•roid•ism

hy•po•per•fu•sion

hy•po•phos•pha•te•mia

hy•po•pla•sia
h. of right ventricle

hy•po•plas•tic left heart syn•drome

hy•po•re•nin•ism

hy•por•rhea

hy•pos•ta•sis

hy•po•stat•ic

hy•po•ten•sion
amiodarone-induced h.
chronic h.
chronic idiopathic orthostatic h.
chronic orthostatic h.
exercise-induced h.

hy•po•ten•sion *(continued)*
hypovolemic h.
idiopathic orthostatic h.
orthostatic h.
postural h.
refractory h.
secondary orthostatic h.
sudden h.
vascular h.
vasovagal h.

hy•po•ten•sive

hy•po•ther•mia
deep h.
profound h.
topical cardiac h.

hy•po•ther•mic

hy•poth•e•sis
cholesterol h.
Gad's h.
inactive X chromosome h.
LDL h.
leading circle h.

hy•poth•e•sis *(continued)*
lipid h.
low-density lipoprotein h.
Lyon h.
monoclonal h.
response-to-injury h.
Starling's h.

hy•po•thy•roid•ism
amiodarone-induced h.

hy•po•ve•nos•i•ty

hy•po•ven•ti•la•tion
alveolar h.

hy•po•vo•le•mia

hy•po•xan•thine

hy•pox•emia
arterial h.

hy•pox•ia
stagnant h.

hy•pox•ic

hys•te•re•sis
stimulation h.

I

I
    inhibited (pacemaker code)
    iodine

I
    electric current

IAB
    intra-aortic balloon

IABP
    intra-aortic balloon pump

ibop•amine

ibu•pro•fen

IC (inductance-capacitance) cir•cuit

ICD
    isocitrate dehydrogenase

ICG
    indocyanine green

ICHD
    Intersociety Commission for Heart Disease

ICHD pace•ma•ker code

ico•sa•no•ic acid

ICS
    intercostal space

ic•tus *pl.* ic•tus
    i. cordis

ICU
    intensive care unit

ida•zox•an

id•io•no•dal

id•io•ven•tric•u•lar

IDL
    intermediate-density lipoprotein

IHSS
    idiopathic hypertrophic subaortic stenosis

Il•o•sone

Ilo•ty•cin

im•age
    color flow velocity i's
    ejection fraction i.
    ejection shell i.
    functional i.
    multiple-gated cardiac blood pool i's
    paradox i.
    parametric i.
    phase i.
    T1 weighted i.
    T2 weighted i.

imag•ing
    acoustic i.
    cardiac magnetic resonance i.
    cine magnetic resonance i.
    color Doppler i.
    color flow i.
    color flow Doppler i.
    CW (continuous wave) Doppler i.
    digital cardiac i.
    dipyridamole thallium i.
    Doppler color flow i.
    Doppler flow i.
    exercise i.
    exercise redistribution thallium-201 i.
    exercise thallium-201 i.
    functional i.
    gated i.
    gated blood pool i.
    gated cardiac blood pool i.
    hot spot i.

imag•ing *(continued)*
- indium-111–labeled platelet i.
- infarct avid i.
- invasive i.
- magnetic resonance i. (MRI)
- mask-mode cardiac i.
- metabolic i.
- multi-gated blood pool i.
- myocardial i.
- myocardial fatty acid i.
- myocardial infarct i.
- myocardial metabolic i.
- myocardial perfusion i.
- noninvasive i.
- nuclear magnetic resonance i.
- planar i.
- planar Tl 201 i.
- proton magnetic resonance i.
- PW (pulsed wave) Doppler i.
- pyrophosphate i.
- pyrophosphate infarct i.
- radionuclide i.
- redistribution i.
- SPECT i.
- SPECT exercise-redistribution thallium i.
- SPECT thallium i.
- stress i.
- stress-redistribution thallium-201 i.
- stress thallium-201 myocardial perfusion i.
- Tc 99m PYP i.
- technetium Tc 99m pyrophosphate i.
- thallium stress i.
- thallium stress-redistribution i.
- thallium-201 i.
- thallium-201 dipyridamole myocardial i.
- thallium-201 planar i.
- thallium-201 SPECT i.

imag•ing *(continued)*
- thallium-201 stress i.
- tomographic i.
- tomographic thallium Tl 201 i.
- transesophageal Doppler color flow i.
- two-dimensional color Doppler i.
- ultrasound i.

im•bal•ance
- acid-base i.

imi•pen•em

imip•ra•mine hy•dro•chlo•ride

im•mune

im•mu•ni•ty
- cell-mediated i.
- humoral i.
- humoral cell–mediated i.

im•mu•no•as•say
- enzyme-linked i.
- fluorescence i.

im•mu•no•de•pres•sion

im•mu•no•de•pres•sive

im•mu•no•dif•fu•sion
- radial i. (RID)

im•mu•no•glob•u•lin

im•mu•no•log•ic

im•mu•no•re•ac•tion

im•mu•no•re•ac•tiv•i•ty

im•mu•no•sup•pres•sant

im•mu•no•sup•pres•sion
- chronic maintenance i.

im•mu•no•sup•pres•sive

im•mu•no•ther•a•py

im•pair•ment
functional aerobic i.

im•pa•ten•cy

im•pa•tent

im•ped•ance
aortic i.
circuit i.
driving i.
polarization i.
sensing i.
source i.
vascular i.

Im•pel•ler pump

im•po•tence

Im•pril

im•pulse
afferent i.
apex i.
apical i.
cardiac i.
episternal i.
left parasternal i's
precordial i.
propagating i.
reentrant i.
right parasternal i's
sinus i.
systolic apical i.

im•pulse gen•er•a•tor

Im•u•ran

In
indium

in•ac•tiv•i•ty
physical i.

in•ci•sion
fish-mouth i.
median sternotomy i.
midline i.
stab i.
thoracotomy i.
transverse i.

in•ci•su•ra *pl.* in•ci•su•rae
i. apicis cordis

in•ci•sure
i. of apex of heart

in•com•pe•tence
aortic i.
i. of the cardiac valves
relative i.
valvular i.

in•con•ti•nen•tia pig•men•ti
syndrome

in•da•cri•none

In•da•meth

in•dap•am•ide

in•dec•ain•ide

In•der•al

in•dex *pl.* in•dex•es, in•di•ces
body mass i.
cardiac i.
cardiac output i.
cardiac risk i.
cardiothoracic i.
diastolic pressure–time i.
ejection phase i.
erythrocyte indices
isovolumetric phase
indices
left ventricular diastolic
phase i.
left ventricular stroke
work i.
oxygen consumption i.
ponderal i.
Quetelet i.
right ventricular stroke
work i.
stroke i.
systolic pressure–time i.
tension-time i.

in•di•ca•tor
Schneider's i.

in•di•um
i.-111
i.-113m

In•do•cid

In•do•cin

in•do•cy•a•nine green

in•do•meth•a•cin
i. sodium

in•farct
anemic i.
brain i.
calcified myocardial i.
embolic i.
hemorrhagic i.
nontransmural i.
pale i.
red i.
subendocardial i.
thrombotic i.
transmural i.

in•farc•tec•to•my

in•farc•tion
anterior myocardial i.
anteroinferior myocardial i.
anterolateral myocardial i.
anteroseptal myocardial i.
atrial i.
atrial myocardial i.
cardiac i.
inferior myocardial i.
inferolateral myocardial i.
lateral myocardial i.
myocardial i.
non-Q-wave i.
posterior myocardial i.
pulmonary i.
Q-wave i.
right ventricular i.
secondary i.
septal myocardial i.
silent myocardial i.
subacute i.

in•farc•tion *(continued)*
subendocardial acute myocardial i.
subendocardial myocardial i.
transmural i.
transmural myocardial i.

in•fec•tion
bacterial i.
cardiac i.
cytomegalovirus i.
fungal i.
metastatic i.
nosocomial i.
respiratory i.
spirochetal i.
systemic i.

in•fec•tive

in•fe•ro•lat•er•al

in•fe•ro•me•di•an

in•fe•ro•pos•te•ri•or

in•fil•tra•tion
adipose i.
fatty i.

in•flam•ma•tion
pericardial i.

in•flu•en•za

in•fra•cla•vic•u•lar

in•fra•cos•tal

in•fra•scap•u•lar

in•fra•ster•nal

In•fu•morph

in•fun•dib•u•lec•to•my
Brock's i.

in•fun•dib•u•lum *pl.* in•fun•dib•u•la
i. of heart

in•fu•sion
bone marrow i.
computerized drug i.

in•hi•bi•tion
myopotential i.
Wedensky i.

in•hib•i•tor
ACE i.
adrenergic i.
angiotensin-converting enzyme (ACE) i's
atriopeptidase i.
carbonic anhydrase i.
converting enzyme i.
cyclooxygenase i.
monoamine oxidase i. (MAOI)
oxysterol i.
phosphodiesterase i.
plasminogen activator i. (PAI)
thromboxane synthase i.

in•jec•tion
intramural i.

in•jec•tor
power i.

in•ju•ry
catecholamine i.
current of i.
diastolic current of i.
ischemic i.
nonpenetrating cardiac i.
penetrating cardiac i.
pseudocurrent of i.
reperfusion i.
systolic current of i.

in-line

in•ner•va•tion
afferent i.
cardiac i.
efferent i.
parasympathetic i.
spinal i.
sympathetic i.
vagal i.

In•no•var

In•o•cor

in•o•sine

in•o•trope

in•o•trop•ic
negatively i.
positively i.

ino•tro•py

in•spi•ra•tion

in•sta•bil•i•ty
electrical i.

in•stru•ment
sternal approximation fixation i.
valve i.
Wolvek sternal approximation fixation i.

in•suf•fi•cien•cy
aortic i.
cardiac i.
cerebrovascular i.
coronary i.
mitral i.
myocardial i.
pulmonary i.
pump i.
traumatic aortic i.
tricuspid i.
i. of the valves
valvular i.

in•su•la•tor
lead i.

in•su•lin
glucose-i.-potassium

in•ten•si•fi•er
cesium iodide image i.
image i.

in•ten•si•ty
point of maximal i.

in•ter•an•nu•lar

in•ter•atri•al

in•ter•au•ric•u•lar

in•ter•cap•il•lary

in•ter•ca•rot•ic

in•ter•ca•rot•id

in•ter•cos•tal

in•ter•de•pen•dence
 ventricular i.

in•ter•face
 electrode-tissue i.

in•ter•fer•ence
 atrioventricular i.
 conducted i.
 electrical i.
 electromagnetic i.
 low-frequency i.
 magnetic i.
 mechanical i.
 microwave i.
 radio-frequency i.

in•ter•fer•on

in•ter•leu•kin
 i.-1 (IL-1)

In•ter•lith pulse generator

In•ter•na•tion•al So•ci•e•ty for Heart and Lung Trans•plan•ta•tion

in•ter•po•lat•ed

in•ter•rup•tion
 inferior vena caval i.

In•ter•so•ci•e•ty Com•mis•sion for Heart Dis•ease

in•ter•val
 A–A i.
 a–c i.
 Ae–H i.
 A–H i.
 atrioventricular i.
 auriculoventricular i.
 automatic pacing i.
 A–V i.
 cardioarterial i.
 coupling i.

in•ter•val *(continued)*
 electromechanical i.
 escape i.
 H–Ae i.
 His-ventricular (H–V) i.
 H–V i.
 interectopic i.
 isovolumetric i.
 magnet pacing i.
 P–A i.
 pacemaker escape i.
 pacing i.
 P–J i.
 postsphygmic i.
 P–P i.
 PQ i.
 P–R i.
 presphygmic i.
 Q–R i.
 QRS i.
 QRST i.
 QS_2 i.
 Q–T i.
 Q–Tc i.
 R–R i.
 S_2-OS i.
 ST i.
 systolic time i.
 total electromechanical i.
 V–A i.
 V–V i.

in•ter•val•vu•lar

in•ter•vas•cu•lar

in•ter•ven•tric•u•lar

in•ti•ma

in•ti•mal

in•ti•mi•tis

in•tol•er•ance
 carbohydrate i.
 glucose i.

in•tox•i•ca•tion
 digitalis i.

in•tra-aor•tic

in•tra-ar•te•ri•al

in•tra-atri•al

in•tra-au•ric•u•lar

In•tra•bu•ta•zone

in•tra•car•di•ac

in•tra•ca•val

in•tra•cav•i•tary

in•tra•cor•dal

in•tra•cor•o•nary

in•tra•mu•ral

in•tra•myo•car•di•al

in•tra•peri•car•di•al

in•tra•tho•rac•ic

in•tra•vas•cu•lar

in•tra•ve•nous

in•tra•ven•tric•u•lar

in•tro•duc•er

In•tro•pin

in•tu•bate

in•tu•ba•tion

in•va•lid•ism
- psychological i.

in•ver•sion
- T wave i.
- visceral i.

io•dine
- i.-123
- lithium-i.
- polyvinylpyrrolidone-i.
- povidone-i.

io•hex•ol

ion
- calcium i.

Io•nes•cu
- I.-Shiley pericardial valve

io•pam•i•dol

io•thal•a•mate
- i. meglumine
- i. sodium

io•ver•sol

iox•a•glate
- i. meglumine
- i. sodium

ipo•date
- i. calcium
- i. sodium

IPPB
- intermittent positive pressure breathing

Ir
- iridium

irid•i•um
- i.-191m
- i.-192
- platinum-i.

iri•do•do•ne•sis

iron
- i. dextran

ir•ra•di•a•tion
- electromagnetic i.
- nuclear i.

ir•reg•u•lar•i•ty
- i. of pulse
- sinus i.

ir•ri•ga•tion

ISA
- intrinsic sympathomimetic activity

is•che•mia
- brachiocephalic i.
- cardiac i.
- cerebral i.
- colonic i.
- exercise-induced regional i.
- gut i.
- myocardial i.

is•che•mia *(continued)*
silent i.

ISD
isosorbide dinitrate

ISDN
isosorbide dinitrate

Is•me•lin

Iso-Bid

iso•ci•trate de•hy•dro•gen•ase (NAD^+)

iso•en•zyme

iso•eth•a•rine
i. hydrochloride
i. mesylate

iso•flu•rane

iso•form

iso•ge•ne•ic

iso•ge•ner•ic

iso•gen•ic

iso•graft

isol•o•gous

Iso•nate

iso•ni•a•zid

iso•plas•tic

iso•pro•te•re•nol
i. hydrochloride
i. sulfate

Isop•tin

Isor•bid

Isor•dil

iso•re•ponse

iso•sor•bide
i. dinitrate
i. mononitrate

Isot•amine

iso•tope
positron-emitting i.
radioactive i.

iso•trans•plan•ta•tion

Iso•trate

iso•tret•i•noin

iso•vo•lum•ic

Iso•vue

iso•zyme

is•ra•di•pine

Is•rael
I. retractor

isth•mus *pl.* is•thmi
i. of aorta
i. aortae
i. of Vieussens

Isu•prel

IV
interventricular
intravascular
intravenous

I-V
intraventricular

IVC
inferior vena cava

IVCD
intraventricular conduction defect
intraventricular conduction delay

IVCP
inferior vena cava pressure

IVCV
inferior venacavography

Ive•mark
I's syndrome
Polhemus-Schafer-I. syndrome

IVP
intravenous push
intraventricular pressure

IVPB
intravenous piggyback

IVS
interventricular septum

IVSD
interventricular septal defect

IWMI
inferior wall myocardial infarction

Izo•nid

J

J
joule

Jac•coud
J's arthritis
J's sign

Jad•as•sohn
nevus sebaceous of J.

James
J. fiber

Jane•way
J. lesion

Jan•i•mine

Ja•quet
J's apparatus

Ja•risch
Bezold-J. reflex

Jar•vik
J. 7 artificial heart

Ja•vid
J. shunt

Jen•kins
J. Activity Survey

Jer•vell
J. and Lange-Nielsen syndrome

John•son
J.-Stevens disease
Stevens-J. syndrome

Jones
J. criteria in rheumatic fever diagnosis

joule

J point

JT
junctional tachycardia

Jud•kins
J. coronary arteriography
J. coronary catheter
J. left coronary arteriography catheter
J. left coronary catheter
J. method
J. pigtail left ventriculography catheter
J. right coronary arteriography catheter
J. right coronary catheter
J. technique

junc•tion
atrioventricular j.
AV j.
gap j.
QRS–ST j.
tight j.

junc•tion•al

jux•ta•car•di•ac

jux•ta•duc•tal

J wave

K
  potassium

Kabi•ki•nase

kal•li•kre•in

Kall•mann
  K's syndrome

kan•a•my•cin
  k. B
  k. sulfate

Kan•trex

ka•o•lin
  k.-pectate

Ka•on

Ka•po•si
  K's sarcoma

Karp
  K. aortic punch

Kar•ta•gen•er
  K's syndrome
  K's triad

Kas•ter
  Lillehei-K. pivoting-disk valve
  Lillehei-K. prosthetic valve

Ka•wa•sa•ki
  K. disease
  K. syndrome

Kay
  K. aorta clamp
  Lambert-K. aorta clamp
  Lambert-K. clamp

Kay•ex•a•late

Kearns
  K.-Sayre syndrome

Kef•let

Kef•lex

Kef•lin

Kef•tab

Kef•zol

Keith
  K's bundle
  K. needle
  K's node
  K.-Flack node
  K.-Wagener-Barker classification

Kel•ly
  K. clamp
  K. hemostat

Ken•my•cin

Kent
  K's bundle
  K.-His bundle

ker•a•tan•sul•fa•tu•ria

Kerck•ring
  nodules of K.

Ker•ley
  K. A lines
  K. B lines

Kes•trin

Kes•trone

Ket•a•lar

keta•mine hy•dro•chlo•ride

keV
  kilo electron volt

key
  Allen k.

kick
  atrial k.

kid•ney
  flea-bitten k.

kid•ney *(continued)*
- Goldblatt k.
- polycystic k.
- unilateral multicystic k.

Kil•lip
- K's classification of heart disease
- K. clinical score

Kim•ray
- K.-Greenfield filter

ki•ne•mia

ki•ne•mic

ki•net•ics
- first-order k.
- myocardial k.
- resting k.
- second order k.
- zero order k.

ki•ne•to•car•dio•gram

ki•ne•to•car•di•og•ra•phy

King•el•la
- *K. kingae*

ki•nin

ki•nin•o•gen
- high molecular weight k.
- low molecular weight k.

Klavi•kor•dal

Kleb•si•el•la
- *K. pneumoniae*

Klein
- Franceschetti-K. syndrome
- K.-Waardenburg syndrome

Klem•per•er
- K's disease

Klip•pel
- K.-Feil sequence

knife
- deep k.
- Lebsche sternal k.
- nerve k.

knife *(continued)*
- skin k.
- sternal k.

knob
- aortic k.

knock
- diastolic pericardial k.
- pericardial k.

knuck•le
- aortic k.

Koch
- K's node

Kö•cher
- K. clamp

Kof•ran•yi
- K.-Michaelis respirometer

Kon•no
- K. procedure
- K.-Sakakibara bioptome

Ko•rán•yi
- K's auscultation
- K's percussion

Korn•zweig
- Bassen-K. syndrome

Ko•rot•koff
- K's method
- K. sounds
- K's test

K-Phen

Krebs
- K. cycle

Krey•sig
- Heim-K. sign
- K's sign

Kru•ken•berg
- K's veins

kryp•ton
- k. Kr 81m

Kuss•maul
- K's disease

Kuss•maul *(continued)*
K's pulse
K's sign
K.-Maier disease

kwash•i•or•kor

ky•mo•gram

ky•mo•graph

ky•mog•ra•phy
roentgen k.

ky•pho•sco•li•o•sis

L

la•bet•a•lol
  l. hydrochloride

lab•o•ra•to•ry
  cardiac catheterization l.
  catheterization l.

la•cer•tus
  l. cordis

lac•tase

lac•tate

L-lac•tate de•hy•dro•gen•ase (LDH)

lac•tic acid

lac•tic de•hy•dro•gen•ase

Lac•to•bac•il•lus

lac•to•syl•cer•a•mide

la•cu•na *pl.* la•cu•nae
  l. vasorum
  l. of vessels

LAD
  left axis deviation

LAD (left anterior descending) ar•te•ry

LAE
  left atrial enlargement

L.A.E. 20

Laën•nec
  L's disease

LAH
  left anterior hemiblock

LAHB
  left anterior hemiblock

LAL (*Limulus* amoebocyte lysate) test

LAMB (lentigenes, atrial myxoma, and blue nevi) syn•drome

Lam•bert
  L.-Kay aorta clamp
  L.-Kay clamp

Lambl
  L's excrescence

lam•i•na *pl.* lam•i•nae
  elastic l., external
  elastic l., internal
  l. parietalis pericardii
  l. visceralis pericardii

Lamy
  Maroteaux-L. mucopolysaccharidosis syndrome

lan•cet

Lan•dis
  Gibbon and L. test

Lan•dou•zy
  L. dystrophy
  L.-Dejerine dystrophy

Lange
  Cornelia de L. syndrome

Lan•gen•beck
  L. retractor

Lange-Niel•sen
  Jervell and L.-N. syndrome

Lan•ger
  L.-Giedion syndrome

Lani•azid

Lano•phyl•lin

la•nos•ter•ol

LAO
  left anterior oblique

LAP
leucine aminopeptidase

lap
laparotomy

La•place
L's law

Lar•gac•til

Lar•o•do•pa

Lar•sen
L's syndrome

lar•va *pl.* lar•vae
l. migrans
visceral l. migrans

la•ser
argon l.
carbon-dioxide l.
CO_2 l.
excimer l.
helium-neon l.
HeNe l.
Nd:YAG l.
neodymium:YAG l.
neodymium:yttrium-aluminum-garnet (Nd:YAG) l.
Yag l.

La•ser•por electrode

La•six

la•ten•cy
pacemaker l.

lat•er•ad

lat•er•al

lat•ero•ab•do•mi•nal

lat•ero•de•vi•a•tion

lat•ero•po•si•tion

Lath•y•rus
L. odoratus

Lau•rence
L.-Biedl syndrome
L.-Moon-Biedl syndrome
L.-Moon-Biedl-Bardet syndrome

law
all-or-none l.
Bowditch's l.
Einthoven l.
Frank's l.
Frank-Starling l.
l. of the heart
Laplace's l.
Marey's l.
Ohm's l.
Starling's l.
Starling's l. of the heart

Lax•o•va
Neu-L. syndrome

lay•er
fascial l.
parietal l. of pericardium
parietal l. of serous pericardium
Purkinje l.
subendocardial l.
subendothelial l.
subepicardial l.
visceral l. of pericardium

LBB
left bundle branch

LBBB
left bundle branch block

LCAD
long chain acyl-CoA dehydrogenase

LCAT
lecithin–cholesterol acyltransferase

LCX (left circumflex) cor•o•nary ar•te•ry

LD
lactate dehydrogenase
lactic dehydrogenase

LDH
lactate dehydrogenase

LDL
low-density lipoprotein

LDL-C
low-density lipoprotein cholesterol

LDLP
low-density lipoprotein

lead
l. apron
l. sulfide

lead
l. I
l. II
l. III
active l.
active fixation l.
l. adaptor
atrial J l.
atrial J-tined l.
augmented unipolar limb l.
aV_F l.
aV_L l.
aV_R l.
bipolar l.
bipolar limb l.
bipolar precordial l.
Bisping l.
chest l.
Christmas tree l.
coaxial l.
coaxial bipolar l.
coil conductor l.
l. connector
corkscrew sutureless l.
coronary sinus l.
crown of thorns l.
DBS l.
drawn–brazed strand (DBS) l.
Dutcher l.
ECG l.
EKG l.

lead *(continued)*
electrocardiogram l.
electrocardiographic l.
endocardial l.
endocardial pacemaker l.
endocardial screw-in l.
epicardial l.
epicardial fishhook l.
epicardial pacemaker l.
esophageal l.
fishhook l.
Frank XYZ l's
hook l.
horizontal plane l.
J l.
limb l's
low impedance l.
magnetic tip l.
Medtronic l.
Medtronic bipolar coaxial atrial J l.
Medtronic multitined pacemaker l.
Medtronic pacemaker l.
Medtronic-Bisping l.
orthogonal l.
Osypka l.
Osypka screw-in l.
pacemaker l.
passive l.
polyurethane l.
precordial l's
quadrifilar l.
ribbon pacemaker l.
right atrial appendage J l.
sagittal l.
screw-in l.
screw-on epicardial pacemaker l.
Siemens-Elema l.
Siemens-Elema pacemaker l.
Siemens-Elema ribbon l.
single-pass dual-chamber l.
stainless steel l.
standard l.
surface l.

lead *(continued)*
- sutureless l.
- temporary pacemaker l.
- three-turn epicardial l.
- three-turn epicardial screw-in l.
- tined l.
- transthoracic l.
- transvenous l.
- transvenous endocardial l.
- transvenous endocardial screw-in l.
- transvenous pacemaker l.
- transverse l.
- unipolar l.
- unipolar augmented limb l.
- unipolar limb l.
- unipolar precordial l.
- V l's
- vertical l.
- wedge tip l.
- Wilson's l's
- l. wire
- X l.
- XYZ l's
- Y l.
- Z l.

leaf•let
- common anterior l.

Lebsche
- L. sternal knife

lec•i•thin

lec•i•thin–cho•les•ter•ol ac•yl•trans•fer•ase (LCAT)

Leff
- L. stethoscope

Le•gio•nel•la

leio•myo•sar•co•ma
- cardiac l.

Lem•li
- Smith-L.-Opitz syndrome

Le•nèg•re
- L's disease

len•tig•i•nes

leo•pard syn•drome

lep•to•spi•ro•sis

Lep•to•trich•ia
- *L. buccalis*

Lerch
- L's percussion

Le•riche
- L's syndrome

le•sion
- atherosclerotic l.
- birds' nest l.
- Bracht-Wächter l.
- Janeway l.
- regurgitant valvular l.

leu•cine am•i•no•pep•ti•dase

leu•ko•cyte
- polymorphonuclear l.

leu•ko•tri•ene

Lev
- L's disease

lev•ar•te•re•nol
- l. bitartrate

Le•vate

Lev•a•tol

lev•el
- isoelectric l.

Le•vine
- L's sign
- Lown-Ganong-L. syndrome

le•vo•car•dia
- isolated l.
- mixed l.

le•vo•do•pa

Lev•o•phed

le•vo•trans•po•si•tion

Lé•vy
Roussy-L. disease
Roussy-L. hereditary areflexic dystasia
Roussy-L. syndrome

Lew•is
L. and Pickering test

LGL (Lown-Ganong-Levine) syndrome

Li
lithium

Lib•man
L.-Sacks disease
L.-Sacks endocarditis
L.-Sacks syndrome

lic•o•rice

li•do•caine
l. hydrochloride

Lie•ber•mann
L.-Burchard reaction
L.-Burchard test

Life Change Units

lift
left parasternal l.

lift•er
vein l.

lig•a•ment
Bérard's l.
l. of Botallo
conus l.
costopericardiac l.
inguinal l.
l. of left superior vena cava
l's of Luschka
pericardiosternal l's
sternopericardiac l's
Teutleben's l's

lig•a•men•tum *pl.* lig•a•men•ta
l. arteriosum

lig•a•men•tum *(continued)*
l. arteriosum arteriae pulmonalis
ligamenta sternopericardiaca
l. venae cavae sinistrae

li•gate

li•ga•tion

lig•a•ture
control l.
distal l.
silk l.
suture l.

Li•kar
Mason-L. limb lead modification

Lil•le•hei
L.-Kaster pivoting-disk valve
L.-Kaster prosthetic valve

limb
anacrotic l.
catacrotic l.

lim•bus *pl.* lim•bi
l. fossae ovalis
l. fossae ovalis [Vieussenii]
l. of Vieussens

lim•it
Nyquist l.

line
arterial l. (A-line)
arterial perfusion l.
central CVP l.
central venous l.
Eberth's l's
isoelectric l.
Kerley A l's
Kerley B l's
median l.
parasternal l.
peripheral CVP l.
pressure l.
pump l.

line *(continued)*
sternal l.
suture l.
venous return l.
Z l.

lin•ea *pl.* lin•eae
l. alba

lin•o•le•ate

lin•o•le•ic acid

lin•o•le•in

lin•o•len•ate

lin•o•len•ic acid

lin•o•lic acid

lip•ac•i•de•mia

lip•ase
acid l.
hepatic l.
hepatic triglyceride l.
lipoprotein l.
pancreatic l.

li•pa•sic

li•pe•mia
l. retinalis

lip•id
l. A
membrane l.
renomedullary l.

Lip•id Re•search Clin•ics Cor•o•nary Pri•mary Pre•ven•tion Tri•al

lip•i•de•mia

lip•id•ic

lip•i•dol•y•sis

lip•i•do•lyt•ic

lip•i•do•sis

lipo•at•ro•phy

lipo•car•di•ac

lipo•cata•bol•ic

lipo•cla•sis

lipo•clas•tic

lipo•cor•ti•coid

lipo•cyte

lipo•di•er•e•sis

lipo•di•er•et•ic

lipo•dys•tro•phia
l. progressiva

lipo•dys•tro•phy
congenital progressive l.
generalized l.
intestinal l.
partial l.
progressive l.
progressive congenital l.
total l.

li•pof•er•ous

lipo•gen•e•sis

lipo•ge•net•ic

lip•o•gen•ic

lipo•gran•u•lo•ma•to•sis
Farber's l.

lip•oid

lip•oi•de•mia

lip•oi•do•sis
arterial l.
cholesterol l.

li•pol•y•sis

lipo•lyt•ic

li•po•ma
cardiac l.

lipo•meta•bol•ic

lipo•me•tab•o•lism

li•pop•a•thy

lipo•pha•gia

lipo•pha•gic

li•poph•a•gy

lipo•phil

lipo•phil•ia

lipo•phil•ic

lipo•poly•sac•cha•ride

lipo•pro•tein
- α-l.
- β-l.
- l. (a)
- alpha l.
- beta l.
- floating beta l's
- high-density l. (HDL)
- intermediate-density l. (IDL)
- low-density l. (LDL)
- Lp(a) l.
- pre-β-l.
- pre-beta l.
- sinking pre-β-l.
- slow pre-β-l.
- very-high-density l. (VHDL)
- very low-density l. (VLDL)
- l. X

lipo•pro•tein•emia

lipo•pro•tein lip•ase
- endothelial l.l.

lipo•sar•co•ma

lipo•some

Li•quae•min

Liq•uid Pred

li•quor *pl.* li•quors, li•quo•res
- l. pericardii

li•sin•o•pril

Li•so•lip•in

lis•sen•ceph•a•ly syndrome

Lis•te•ria
- *L. monocytogenes*

Lith•ane

lith•i•um
- l. chloride

Lith•i•zine

Lith•o•bid

litho•cho•late

litho•cho•lic acid

litho•cho•lyl•gly•cine

litho•cho•lyl•tau•rine

Lith•o•nate

Lith•o•tabs

Lit•ten
- L's diaphragm phenomenon
- L's sign

Lit•tle
- L's disease
- L's syndrome

Lit•wak
- L. mitral valve scissors

Lix•o•lin

LLAT
- left lateral

load•ing
- relaxation l.
- volume l.

Lob•stein
- L's disease

lo•fex•i•dine
- l. hydrochloride

Löff•ler
- L's disease
- L's endocarditis
- L's parietal fibroplastic endocarditis

log•ic
- dual chamber l.

long chain ac•yl-CoA de•hy•dro•gen•ase

Lo•ni•ten

loop
- Gerdy's interarticular l.
- Gerdy's interauricular l.
- Henle's l.
- memory l.
- P l.
- pressure-volume l.
- QRS l.
- T l.
- ventricular pressure-volume l.

Lo•pid

Lo•pre•sor *(Can.)*

Lo•pres•sor *(U.S.)*
- L. HCT

lor•a•ze•pam

lor•cai•nide hy•dro•chlo•ride

Lo•rel•co

Los An•ge•les Heart Stu•dy

lov•a•sta•tin

Low•er
- L's rings
- L's tubercle

Lown
- L.-Ganong-Levine (LGL) syndrome

Low•ry
- Coffin-L. syndrome

Lo•zide

Lo•zol

Lp(a)
- Lp(a) lipoprotein

LPA
- left pulmonary artery

LPH
- left posterior hemiblock

LPHB
- left posterior hemiblock

LPL
- lipoprotein lipase

LPO
- left posterior oblique

LPS
- lipopolysaccharide

LpX
- LpX lipoprotein

LSU
- Life Support Unit

lubb

lubb-dupp

Lu•bin
- Goodale-L. catheter

Lu•di•o•mil

Lud•wig
- L's ganglia
- L's plane

Luer-Lok needle tip

lu•men *pl.* lu•mi•na

lung
- cardiac l.
- pump l.
- shock l.

lu•nu•la *pl.* lu•nu•lae
- lunulae of aortic valves
- lunulae of pulmonary trunk valves
- lunulae of semilunar valves
- lunulae of semilunar valves of aorta
- lunulae valvularum semilunarium aortae
- lunulae valvularum semilunarium trunci pulmonalis

lu·pus
l. erythematosus (LE)
systemic l. erythematosus

Lusch·ka
ligaments of L.

Lu·tem·bach·er
L's complex
L's disease
L's syndrome

LV
left ventricle

LVAD
left ventricular assist device

LVEDP
left ventricular end-diastolic pressure

LVEDV
left ventricular end-diastolic volume

LVEF
left ventricular ejection fraction

LVET
left ventricular ejection time

LVH
left ventricular hypertrophy

LVP
left ventricular pressure

LVS
left ventricular strain

LVSP
left ventricular systolic pressure

LVSV
left ventricular stroke volume

LVSW
left ventricular stroke work

LVSWI
left ventricular stroke work index

LVW
left ventricular work

LVWI
left ventricular work index

17,20-ly·ase

Lyme disease

lym·phad·e·nop·a·thy
immunoblastic l.

lym·phan·gi·o·ma
cardiac l.

lym·pho·cyte

lym·pho·cy·to·tox·ic

lym·pho·ma
B cell l.
non-Hodgkin's l's

lym·pho·sar·co·ma
cardiac l.

lym·pho·tox·in

Ly·on
L. hypothesis

Ly·pho·cin

M

M
multiprogrammable (pacemaker code)

m
milli-

μ
micro-
micron

μA
microampere

Mc·Ar·dle
M's disease
M's syndrome

Mac·Cal·lum
M's patch

Mc·Cune
Albright-M.-Sternberg syndrome
M.-Albright syndrome

Mc·Ginn
M.-White sign

Ma·cha·do
M. test
M.-Guerreiro test

ma·chine
heart-lung m.

mac·ro·re·en·try

mac·ro·shock

Mac·ro·tec

Mag·na·prin

mag·ne·si·um
m. sulfate

mag·ne·to·car·dio·graph

Ma·haim
M. fibers

Mah·ler
M's sign

Mai·er
Kussmaul-M. disease

mal·a·die
m. de Roger

ma·late de·hy·dro·gen·ase

mal·for·ma·tion
cardiac m.

ma·lig·nant

Mal·linc·krodt
M. right-sided double-lumen tube

Mal·lory
M.-Weiss syndrome

mal·nu·tri·tion
protein-calorie m.

ma·neu·ver
Heimlich m.
Müller's m.
Valsalva's m.

man·ga·nese

man·i·fold

man·ni·tol
m. hexanitrate

ma·nom·e·ter

mano·met·ric

MAOI
monoamine oxidase inhibitor

MAP
mean arterial pressure

map
bull's-eye polar coordinate m.
electrophysiologic m.

map *(continued)*
endocardial isochronous m.
polar m.

map•ping
body surface m.
cardiac m.
color Doppler m.
color flow m.
direct cardiac m.
Doppler color flow m.
Doppler flow m.
epicardial m.
epimyocardial m.
intraoperative epicardial m.
retrograde atrial m.
ventricular m.

Ma•prin

ma•pro•ti•line
m. hydrochloride

ma•ras•mus

Mar•che•sa•ni
M's syndrome
Weill-M. syndrome

Ma•rey
M's law

Mar•fan
M's syndrome

mar•gin
right m. of heart

mar•go *pl.* mar•gi•nes
m. dexter cordis

Ma•rie
Charcot-M.-Tooth disease

mar•i•jua•na

Ma•ro•teaux
M.-Lamy mucopolysaccharidosis syndrome

Mar•shall
M's fold

Mar•shall *(continued)*
M's oblique vein
vein of M.
vestigial fold of M.

Mar•tin
M. forceps
M. needle

Mar•tor•ell
M's syndrome

Ma•son
M.-Likar limb lead modification

mass
intracardiac m.
myocardial m.

mas•sage
cardiac m.
carotid sinus m.
closed-chest cardiac m.
heart m.
open-chest cardiac m.

Mas•ter
M. step test
M. two-step exercise test
M. two-step fitness test

MAT
multifocal atrial tachycardia

Mat•as
M. band
M. operation
M. test

match•ing
afterload m.
cross m.

Mat•son
M. rib stripper

Max•air

May•er
M. waves

Ma•yo
- M. clamp
- curved M. scissors
- M. hemostat
- M. needle
- M. scissors
- M. stand

Ma•ze•pine

μC
- microcoulomb

MCH
- mean corpuscular hemoglobin

MCHC
- mean corpuscular hemoglobin concentration

mCi
- millicurie

MCV
- mean corpuscular volume

Mead•ox
- M.-Gabbay unicusp pericardial valve

mech•a•nism
- bronchoconstrictor m.
- compensatory m.
- escape m.
- Frank-Starling m.
- leading circle m.
- reentrant m.
- Starling m.

Meck•el
- M's syndrome
- M.-Gruber syndrome

me•di•as•ti•no•peri•car•di•tis

me•di•as•ti•not•o•my

me•di•as•ti•num *pl.* me•di•as•ti•na
- anterior m.
- inferior m.

me•di•as•ti•num *(continued)*
- middle m.
- posterior m.
- superior m.

me•dio•ne•cro•sis
- m. of aorta

me•di•um *pl.* me•dia, me•di•ums
- contrast m.
- iso-osmolar contrast m.
- isoviscous contrast m.
- radiocontrast m.

Med•ra•lone

Med•rol

Med•tron•ic
- M. bipolar coaxial atrial J lead
- M. connector
- M. multitined pacemaker lead
- M. pacemaker lead
- M. Xyrel pulse generator
- M.-Hall prosthetic valve
- M.-Hall tilting-disk valve

me•dul•la *pl.* me•dul•lae
- adrenal m.

mega•car•dia

Mega•cil•lin

meg•al•gia

meg•a•lo•car•dia

Meigs
- M. capillaries

Mel•la•ril

mem•brane
- alveolar-capillary m.
- alveolocapillary m.
- atrial m.
- Bichat's m.
- cell m.
- cuprophane m.
- elastic m., external

mem•brane *(continued)*
elastic m., internal
fenestrated m.
Gore-Tex surgical m.
Henle's elastic m.
Henle's fenestrated m.
polyacrylonitrile m.
Traube's m.

Men•del•sohn
M's test

Men•est

men•in•gi•tis *pl.* men•in•git•i•des

me•nin•go•coc•cus *pl.* me•nin•go•coc•ci

meno•pause
premature m.

me•per•i•dine hy•dro•chlo•ride

Me•pro•lone

me•ral•lu•ride

mer•cap•to•mer•in
m. sodium

Mer•cu•hy•drin

mer•cu•ry
m.-195m

mero•di•a•stol•ic

mero•myo•sin

Mer•si•lene
M. suture

mes•ar•ter•itis
Mönckeberg's m.

mes•en•chy•mo•ma

meso-aor•ti•tis
m. syphilitica

meso•car•dia

meso•car•di•um
arterial m.

meso•car•di•um *(continued)*
venous m.

meso•ca•val

meso•di•a•stol•ic

meso•phle•bi•tis

meso•sys•tol•ic

meso•the•li•o•ma

MET
metabolic equivalents system

met
metabolic equivalents system

met•a•bol•ic

me•tab•o•lism
cardiac m.
glucose m.
HEP m.
high energy phosphate m.
myocardial m.
pyruvate m.

Meta•hy•drin

met•al
heavy m.
trace m.

meta•mor•pho•sis
fatty m.

meta•pro•ter•e•nol

meta•ram•i•nol
m. bitartrate

met•ar•te•ri•ole

me•tas•ta•sis
cardiac m.
crossed m.

me•ter
Bentley Oxy-State M.
metabolic rate m.

meth•a•cho•line
m. bromide

meth•a•cho•line *(continued)*
m. chloride

met•he•mo•glo•bin•emia

meth•i•cil•lin so•di•um

meth•od
Autenrieth and Funk's m.
Bloor, Pelkan, and Allen's m.
caliper m.
continuous Fick m.
direct Fick m.
direct Fick oxygen uptake m.
Douglas bag m.
dye dilution m.
edge-based detection m.
Eggleston's m.
Fick m.
Fick oxygen m.
gated blood pool m.
indicator dilution m.
indocyanine green dye m.
Judkins m.
Korotkoff's m.
Orsi-Grocco m.
oxygen Fick m.
polarographic m.
rebreathing Fick m.
region integration m.
Sheehan and Dodge m.
sliding scale m.
thermal dilution m.
thermodilution m.

meth•o•hex•i•tal

meth•o•trex•ate
m. sodium

me•thox•amine hy•dro•chlo•ride

meth•oxy•iso•bu•tyl
m. isonitrile

meth•y•clo•thi•a•zide

meth•yl•do•pa

meth•yl•phen•i•date hy•dro•chlo•ride

meth•yl•pred•nis•o•lone
m. aceponate
m. acetate
m. hemisuccinate
m. sodium phosphate
m. sodium succinate
m. suleptanate

meth•yl•xan•thine

meth•y•ser•gide
m. maleate

Met•i•cor•ten

Me•ti•zol

met•o•cu•rine io•dide

me•tol•a•zone

me•to•pro•lol
m. tartrate

Met•ric 21

me•triz•a•mide

Me•tro

me•tro•ni•da•zole
m. hydrochloride

Me•tu•bine

Met•zen•baum
M. scissors

MeV
megaelectron volt

Mev•a•cor

Me•val

me•val•o•nate

me•va•lon•ic acid

me•vino•lin

Mex•ate

mex•il•e•tine
m. hydrochloride

Mex•i•til

Mg
magnesium

mg
milligram

MHC
major histocompatibility complex

MH (Medtronic-Hall) prosthetic valve

MI
myocardial infarction

MIBI
methoxyisobutyl isonitrile

Mi•chae•lis
Kofranyi-M. respirometer

mi•con•a•zole ni•trate

mi•cran•gi•um

mi•cro•am•pere

mi•cro•an•eu•rysm

mi•cro•an•gio•path•ic

mi•cro•an•gi•op•a•thy
thrombotic m.

mi•cro•an•gi•os•co•py

mi•cro•bub•ble

mi•cro•car•dia

mi•cro•cav•i•tary

mi•cro•cir•cuit

mi•cro•cir•cuit•ry

mi•cro•cir•cu•la•tion

mi•cro•cir•cu•la•to•ry

mi•cro•cou•lomb

mi•cro•cu•rie

mi•cro•dis•lodge•ment

mi•cro•dis•place•ment

mi•cro•em•bo•lism
cholesterol m.

mi•cro•em•bo•lus *pl.* mi•cro•em•bo•li

mi•cro•in•farct
focal m.

mi•cro•joule

Mi•cro•nor

mi•cro•par•ti•cle
radiolabeled m.

mi•cro•phone
cardiac catheter-m.

mi•cro•re•en•try

mi•cro•shock

mi•cro•sphere
radiolabeled m's

mi•cro•sphyg•mia

mi•cro•sphyg•my

mi•cro•sur•gery
laser m.
mechanical m.

mi•cro•throm•bo•sis

mi•cro•throm•bus *pl.* mi•cro•throm•bi

mi•cro•vas•cu•lar

mi•cro•vas•cu•la•ture

mid•myo•car•di•al

mid-di•as•to•le

mid-di•as•tol•ic

Mi•da•mor

mid•az•o•lam

mid•sys•to•le

mid•sys•tol•ic

mid•sys•tol•ic click syn•drome

MILIS (Multicenter Investigation for the Limitation of Infarct Size) trial

Mil•ler
- M. syndrome
- M.-Dieker syndrome

mil•li•cu•rie

mil•li•rad

mil•li•rem

Mil•ner
- M. needle

mil•ri•none

min•er•alo•cor•ti•coid

Mini•press

Min•i•tec

Min•i•tran

Mi•not
- M.-von Willebrand syndrome

mi•nox•i•dil

mio•car•dia

Mir•a•don

mis•match•ing
- afterload m.

mi•to•gen

mi•to•my•cin

mi•to•xan•trone
- m. hydrochloride

mi•tral

Mix•ter
- M. clamp

μJ
- microjoule

mL
- milliliter

ml
- milliliter

μm
- micrometer

M-mode

M-mode echo•car•di•og•ra•phy

Mn
- manganese

Mo
- molybdenum

Mo•bin
- M.-Uddin filter
- M.-Uddin filter system

Mo•bitz
- M. atrioventricular block
- M. block
- M. heart block
- M. phenomenon
- M. second degree heart block
- M. type I block
- M. type I second degree heart block
- M. type II block
- M. type II second degree heart block

mode
- committed pacing m.
- fixed rate m.
- gated list m.
- inhibited pacing m.
- magnet pacing m.
- noncommitted pacing m.
- overdrive m.
- triggered m.
- triggered pacing m.

mod•el
- figure-of-eight m.
- Hodgkin-Huxley m.
- leading circle m.
- nonlinear dynamic m.
- ring m.

mod•i•fi•ca•tion
  Mason-Likar limb lead m.

mol•e•cule
  neural cell adhesion m.

mo•lyb•den•um

mo•ment
  magnetic m.

Möncke•berg
  M's arteriosclerosis
  M's calcification
  M's degeneration
  M's mesarteritis
  M's sclerosis

Mon•dor
  M's disease

Mon•ge
  M's disease

Mo•ni•stat

Mon•i•tan

mon•i•tor
  blood gas and chemistry m.
  Holter m.

mon•i•tor•ing
  ambulatory m.
  hemodynamic m.
  Holter m.
  invasive hemodynamic m.
  transtelephone m.
  transtelephonic electrocardiographic m.

Mon•ne•ret
  M's pulse

mono•ac•yl•glyc•er•ol

mono•amine ox•i•dase

mono•car•dio•gram

mono•clo•nal

mono•cro•ta•line

mono•crot•ic

mo•noc•ro•tism

mono•cyte

mono•glyc•er•ide

mono•nu•cle•o•sis
  infectious m.

mono•so•my
  9p m.

Moon
  Laurence-M.-Biedl syndrome
  Laurence-M.-Biedl-Bardet syndrome

Mo•rax•el•la

Mor•gag•ni
  M's nodules
  M.-Adams-Stokes syndrome
  sinus of M.

mor•i•ci•zine

mor•phine

Mor•phi•tec

mor•phol•o•gy
  cardiac m.

Mor•quio
  M's disease
  M's syndrome
  M.-Ullrich syndrome

M.O.S.

Mos•cho•witz
  M's disease
  M's sign
  M's test

Mo•ti•li•um

motion
  diastolic m.
  left ventricular wall m.
  precordial m.
  systolic m.
  systolic anterior m. (SAM)
  ventricular wall m.

motion *(continued)*
wall m.

move•ment
circus m.

mox•a•lac•tam
m. disodium

Mox•am

MPI DTPA

MPI MAA

MPI Py•ro•phos•phate

MR
magnetic resonance
mitral regurgitation

MRC
Medical Research Council

MRFIT
Multiple Risk Factor Intervention Trial

MRI
magnetic resonance imaging

M S Con•tin

msec
millisecond

MSIR

mt
mitochondria

mu•co•lip•i•do•sis
m. III

mu•co•poly•sac•cha•ri•do•sis
m. I H
m. IH/S
m. IS
m. IV
m. VI
m. VII

Mu•cor

mu•cro *pl.* mu•cro•nes
m. cordis

MUGA (multiple gated acquisition) scan

Mül•ler
M's experiment
M's maneuver
M's sign

mul•ti•fi•lar

mul•ti•fo•cal

mul•ti•form

mul•ti•gat•ed

mul•ti•pha•sic

mul•ti•ple len•ti•gines syn•drome

Mul•ti•ple Risk Fac•tor In•ter•ven•tion Tri•al (MRFIT)

mul•ti•pli•er
voltage m.

mul•ti•ves•sel

Mu•ret
Quénu-M. sign

mur•mur
accidental m.
anemic m.
aneurysmal m.
aortic m.
aortic diastolic m.
aortic systolic m.
apex m.
apical m.
apical diastolic m's
apical mid-diastolic m.
apical mid-diastolic heart m.
apical systolic heart m.
arterial m.
atrioventricular flow rumbling m.
atrioventricular flow rumbling heart m.
attrition m.
Austin Flint m.
basal diastolic m's

mur•mur *(continued)*
basal systolic m.
bellows m.
blood m.
brain m.
cardiac m.
cardiopulmonary m.
cardiorespiratory m.
Carey Coombs m.
carotid artery m.
continuous m.
continuous heart m.
cooing m.
crescendo m.
Cruveilhier-Baumgarten m.
decrescendo m.
diamond-shaped m.
diamond-shaped ejection m.
diamond-shaped holosystolic m.
diastolic m.
diastolic diminuendo m.
diastolic heart m.
ductus m.
Duroziez's m.
early diastolic m.
early diastolic blowing m.
early systolic m.
early systolic ejection m.
early systolic heart m.
ejection m.
ejection systolic m.
extracardiac m.
Flint's m.
friction m.
functional m.
functional heart m.
functional mitral diastolic m.
Gibson m.
Graham Steell's m.
groaning m.
Hamman's m.
heart m.
hemic m.
holosystolic m.

mur•mur *(continued)*
holosystolic heart m.
hourglass m.
humming-top m.
incidental m.
innocent m.
innocent systolic ejection m.
inorganic m.
intracardiac m.
late apical systolic m.
late diastolic m.
late systolic m.
late systolic heart m.
machinery m.
mid-diastolic m.
mid-diastolic heart m.
mid-diastolic rumbling m.
midsystolic m.
midsystolic aortic m.
midsystolic ejection m.
midsystolic heart m.
midsystolic pulmonic m.
midsystolic systolic m.
mitral m.
mitral diastolic m.
mitral regurgitant m.
musical m.
nonholosystolic regurgitant m.
nonorganic mitral diastolic m.
normal m.
organic m.
pansystolic m.
pansystolic apical m.
patent ductus arteriosus m.
pericardial m.
physiologic m.
physiological midsystolic m.
pleuropericardial m.
prediastolic m.
presystolic m.
presystolic crescendo m.
pulmonic m.
pulmonic systolic m.

mur•mur *(continued)*
regurgitant m.
regurgitant systolic m.
Roger's m.
rumbling m.
sea-gull m.
seesaw m.
Steell's m.
stenosal m.
stenotic m.
Still's m.
subclavicular m.
systolic m.
systolic heart m.
to-and-fro m.
Traube's m.
tricuspid m.
tricuspid regurgitant m.
twanging string m.
vascular m.
venous m.
ventricular filling m.
ventricular filling heart m.
vibratory systolic m.

Mur•phy
M's percussion
M. retractor

mus•cle
cardiac m.
intercostal m.
papillary m's
papillary m. of conus arteriosus
papillary m. of left ventricle, anterior
papillary m. of left ventricle, posterior
papillary m. of right ventricle, anterior
papillary m. of right ventricle, posterior
papillary m's of right ventricle, septal
pectinate m's
pectoralis major m.
skeletal m's
subepicardial m.

mus•cu•lus *pl.* mus•cu•li
musculi papillares
m. papillaris anterior ventriculi dextri
m. papillaris anterior ventriculi sinistri
m. papillaris posterior ventriculi dextri
m. papillaris posterior ventriculi sinistri
musculi papillares septales ventriculi dextri
musculi pectinati

Mus•set
M's sign

Mus•tard
M. atrial switch procedure
M. interatrial baffle
M. operation
M. technique

Mu•ta•my•cin

MVO_2
myocardial oxygen consumption

$M\dot{V}O_2$
myocardial oxygen consumption

MVP
mitral valve prolapse

My•am•bu•tol

my•as•the•nia
angiosclerotic m.
m. gravis

My•co•bac•te•ri•um
M. chelonei
M. fortuitum
M. tuberculosis

My•co•plas•ma
M. pneumoniae

my•cot•ic

My-E

my•ec•to•my

My•krox

Myl•er•an

My•meth•a•sone

myo•atri•al

myo•car•di•ac

myo•car•di•al

myo•car•dio•gram

myo•car•dio•graph

myo•car•di•ol•y•sis

myo•car•di•op•a•thy
alcoholic m.
chagasic m.

myo•car•di•or•rha•phy

myo•car•di•o•sis

myo•car•dit•ic

myo•car•di•tis
acute bacterial m.
acute isolated m.
bacterial m.
chronic m.
diphtheritic m.
fibrous m.
Fiedler's m.
fragmentation m.
fungal m.
giant cell m.
hypersensitivity m.
idiopathic m.
infectious m.
infective m.
interstitial m.
metazoal m.
parenchymatous m.
protozoal m.
rheumatic m.
rheumatoid m.
rickettsial m.
spirochetal m.
toxic m.
tuberculoid m.

myo•car•di•tis *(continued)*
tuberculous m.
viral m.

myo•car•di•um
hibernating m.
ischemic m.
stunned m.
unstable m.

myo•car•do•sis

myo•cyte
Anichkov's m.
atrial m.
ventricular m.

myo•cy•tol•y•sis
coagulative m.
focal m. of heart

myo•ede•ma

myo•en•do•car•di•tis

myo•fas•ci•al

myo•fi•bril

myo•fi•bril•lar ATP•ase

myo•fi•bro•blast
contractile m.

myo•fi•bro•sis
m. cordis

myo•fila•ment

myo•glo•bin

my•ol•y•sis
m. cardiotoxica

myo•ne•cro•sis
clostridial m.

myo•path•ia
m. cordis

my•op•a•thy
centronuclear m.
myotubular m.
nemaline m.

myo•peri•car•di•tis

myo•po•ten•tial

my•o•sin
    cardiac m.

my•o•sin ATP•ase

myo•si•tis

my•ot•o•my

myo•to•nia
    m. congenita

myr•is•tate

my•ris•tic acid

My•ro•sem•ide

Myth•ro•my•cin

myx•ede•ma

myx•o•ma *pl.* myx•o•mas, myx•o•ma•ta
    atrial m.
    cardiac m.
    complex cardiac m.
    familial cardiac m.
    intracardiac m.
    sporadic cardiac m.
    ambulatory ECG m.

N

N
  nitrogen

Na
  sodium

na•do•lol

Naf•cil

naf•cil•lin
  n. sodium

Na•ger
  N. acrofacial dysostosis syndrome

Nal•crom

Nall•pen

nal•ox•one hy•dro•chlo•ride

NAME (nevi, atrial myxoma, myxoid neurofibroma, ephelides) syn•drome

na•nism
  mulibrey n.

Nap•trate

Na•qua

Nar•can

nar•cot•ic

NASPE spe•cif•ic code

Na•than
  N. pacemaker

Na•tion•al Cho•les•ter•ol Ed•u•ca•tion Pro•gram

Na•tion•al Heart, Lung, and Blood In•sti•tute

Na•tion•al In•sti•tutes of Health

na•tre•mia

na•tri•ure•sis

na•tri•uret•ic

Nat•ure•tin

Naugh•ton
  N. cardiac exercise treadmill
  N. protocol
  N. test
  N. treadmill protocol

nau•sea

NBG pace•maker code

Nd
  neodymium

Nd:Yag (neodymium:yttrium-aluminum-garnet) la•ser

Ne
  neon

Neb•cin

ne•cro•sis *pl.* ne•cro•ses
  arteriolar n.
  coagulation n.
  cystic medial n.
  Erdheim's cystic medial n.
  medial n.
  myocardial n.
  renal cortical n.
  selective myocardial cell n.
  tubular n.

nee•dle
  aneurysm n.
  arteriogram n.
  atraumatic n.
  blunt point n.
  conventional cutting n.
  Cope's n.
  Cournand n.
  curved n.
  cutting n.
  Deschamps' n.
  diamond point n.

nee•dle *(continued)*
elliptical eye n.
eyeless n.
Fergie n.
Ferguson n.
French eye n.
hypodermic n.
inverted cutting n.
Keith n.
ligature n.
Martin n.
Mayo n.
Milner n.
precision point n.
reverse cutting n.
spatula n.
spinal n.
square eye n.
straight n.
surgeon's regular n.
suture n.
suture-release n.
swaged n.
taper n.
taper point n.
Tapercut n.
transseptal n.
trocar n.

nee•dle hold•er
Crile-Wood n.h.
Heaney n.h.
Rogers n.h.
Stratte n.h.

NEFA
nonesterified fatty acids

Neis•se•ria
N. meningitidis

Nel•son
N. scissors

Nem•bu•tal

Neo-Co•de•ma

neo•dym•i•um

Neo-Es•trone

Neo-Met•ric

neo•my•cin

ne•on

Neo•sar

Neo•scan

neo•stig•mine

Neo-Sy•neph•rine

neo•vas•cu•lar•iza•tion

ne•phri•tis *pl.* ne•phrit•i•des
familial n.

neph•ro•car•di•ac

ne•phrop•a•thy
analgesic n.
diabetic n.

neph•ro•tox•ic•i•ty

Neph•rox

NERICP
New England Regional Infant Cardiac Program

Nernst
N. equation

nerve
accelerator n's
cardiac n., cervical, inferior
cardiac n's
cardiac n., cervical, middle
cardiac n., cervical, superior
cardiac n., inferior
cardiac n., middle
cardiac n., superior
cardiac n's, supreme
cardiac n's, thoracic
depressor n.
parasympathetic n.
phrenic n.
tenth cranial n.
vagus n.
vasoconstrictor n.

nerve *(continued)*
vasodilator n.
vasomotor n.

ner•vus *pl.* ner•vi
n. cardiacus cervicalis inferior
n. cardiacus cervicalis medius
n. cardiacus cervicalis superior
n. cardiacus inferior
n. cardiacus medius
n. cardiacus superior
nervi cardiaci thoracici

nest
birds' n's

net
Trolard's n.

net•il•mi•cin sul•fate

Ne•tro•my•cin

net•work
Chiari's n.
Purkinje's n.
subendocardial terminal n.
venous n.

Neu
N.-Laxova syndrome

neu•ral

neu•ral•gia
glossopharyngeal n.

neu•ro•blas•to•ma

neu•ro•car•di•ac

neu•ro•cir•cu•la•to•ry

neu•ro•fi•bro•ma
cardiac n.

neu•ro•fi•bro•ma•to•sis

neu•ro•fi•bro•ma•to•sis syn•drome

neu•ro•lep•tic

Neu•ro•lon
N. suture

neu•ro•mod•u•la•tor

neu•ro•my•op•a•thy

neu•rop•a•thy

neu•ro•pep•tide
n. tyrosine

neu•ro•ple•gia

neu•ro•sis *pl.* neu•ro•ses
anxiety n.

neu•rot•i•cism

neu•ro•trans•mit•ter

neu•tron

neu•tro•pe•nia

neu•tro•phil

ne•vus *pl.* ne•vi
n. sebaceus of Jadassohn

New York Heart As•so•ci•a•tion

New York Heart As•so•ci•a•tion (NYHA) clas•si•fi•ca•tion

nex•us *pl.* nex•us

NHLBI
National Heart, Lung & Blood Institute

NH re•gion

Ni
nickel

Nia-Bid

Ni•ac

Ni•a•cels

ni•a•cin

ni•car•di•pine
n. hydrochloride

nick•el
n.-cadmium

Nico-400

Nic•o•bid

Ni•co•la•do•ni
N's sign
N.-Branham sign

Nic•o•lar

Nic•o•tin•ex

nic•o•tin•ic acid

ni•fed•i•pine

NIH
National Institutes of Health

Ni•lor•ic

Ni•ong

Nip•ride

ni•trate

ni•trite
amyl n.

Ni•tro-Bid

Ni•tro•cap

Ni•tro•cine

Ni•tro•disc

Ni•tro-Dur

Ni•tro•gard

ni•tro•gen
n.-13
n.-13 ammonia
n.-13 ammonium

ni•tro•glyc•er•in
topical n.
transdermal n.

Ni•tro•glyn

Ni•tro•ject

Ni•trol

Ni•tro•lin

Ni•tro•lin•gual

Ni•tro•net

Ni•trong

Ni•tro•press

ni•tro•prus•side
sodium n.

Ni•tro•span

Ni•tro•stat

NK (natural killer) cell

NMR
nuclear magnetic resonance

No•car•dia
N. israelii

noc•tu•ria

node
Aschoff's n.
n. of Aschoff and Tawara
atrioventricular n.
AV n.
compact atrioventricular (AV) n.
Flack's n.
Koch's n.
lymph n.
Osler's n's
SA n.
sinoatrial n.
sinuatrial n.
sinus n.
n. of Tawara

no•do•ven•tric•u•lar

nod•ule
Albini's n's
n's of aortic valve
n's of Arantius
Aschoff's n's
Bianchi's n's
n's of Kerckring
Morgagni's n's

nod•ule *(continued)*
  n's of pulmonary trunk valves
  subcutaneous n.

nod•u•lus *pl.* nod•u•li
  noduli valvularum semilunarium

no•dus *pl.* no•di
  n. atrioventricularis
  n. sinuatrialis

non•ath•er•o•ma•tous

non•ath•ero•scle•rot•ic

non•car•dio•gen•ic

non•com•pen•sa•tory

non•com•pli•ance

non•gly•co•side

non•in•farc•tion

non•rheu•mat•ic

Noo•nan
  N's syndrome

No•Pro•file
  N. balloon catheter

nor•adren•a•line
  n. bitartrate

nor•epi•neph•rine
  n. bitartrate

nor•eth•in•drone
  n. acetate

Nor•lu•tate

Nor•lu•tin

nor•mo•cal•ce•mia

nor•mo•cal•ce•mic

nor•mo•cho•les•ter•ol•emia

nor•mo•cho•les•ter•ol•emic

Nor•mo•dyne

nor•mo•lip•i•de•mia

nor•mo•lip•i•de•mic

nor•mo•ten•sion

nor•mo•ten•sive

nor•mo•ther•mia

nor•mo•ther•mic

Nor•pace

Nor•pram•in

Nor-Q.D.

nor•trip•ty•line hy•dro•chlo•ride

notch
  a n.
  aortic n.
  dicrotic n.
  incisural n.
  Sibson's n.
  sternal n.

No•va•mox•in

No•van•trone

No•vo Am•pi•cil•lin

No•vo•bu•ta•zone

No•vo•car•ba•maz

No•vo-Chlor•pro•ma•zine

No•vo•ci•me•tine

No•vo•clox•in

No•vo•di•pam

No•vo•fi•brate

No•vo•flu•pam

No•vo-Hy•dra•zide

No•vo-Hy•la•zin

No•vo•lex•in

No•vo•lo•ra•zem

No•vo•me•do•pa

No•vo•meth•a•cin

No•vo•me•to•prol

No•vo•ni•da•zol

No•vo-Ni•fed•in

No•vo•pra•mine

No•vo•pran•ol

No•vo•py•ra•zone

No•vo•re•ser•pine

No•vo•ryth•ro

No•vo•sal•mol

No•vo•sem•ide

No•vo•sor•bide

No•vo•sox•a•zole

No•vo•spi•ro•ton

No•vo-Sun•dac

No•vo-Tha•li•done

No•vo•tri•mel

No•vo•tri•o•lam

No•vo•trip•tyn

No•vo-Ver•a•mil

No•vox•a•pam

NPC
  nodal premature complex

NPO
  L. nil per os (nothing by mouth)

NPY
  neuropeptide tyrosine

N re•gion

NSR
  normal sinus rhythm

NS-ST
  nonspecific ST segment

NS-ST-T
  nonspecific ST segment and T wave

NS-T
  nonspecific T wave

NT
  nodal tachycardia

NTP
  sodium nitroprusside

NTS

nu•cle•ar

nu•clide

Nu-Lo•raz

num•ber
  Euler n.

Ny•core pigtail catheter

Ny•dra•zid

NYHA
  New York Heart Association

Ny•quist
  N. frequency
  N. limit

O

O
- none (pacemaker code)
- oxygen

Ω
- ohm

obe•si•ty-hy•po•ven•ti•la•tion syn•drome

ob•struc•tion
- atrial o.
- coronary o.
- left ventricular outflow o.
- pulmonary vascular o.
- pulmonary venous o.
- right ventricular o.
- right ventricular outflow o.
- subpulmonic o.
- subvalvular o.

ob•tu•ra•tor
- Carpentier tricuspid o.

oc•clud•er
- balloon o.
- Hunter detachable balloon o.
- tilting-disk o.

oc•clu•sion
- acute thrombotic o.
- coronary o.

ochro•no•sis

Ochs•ner
- O. clamp

oc•ta•dec•a•no•ate

oc•ta•de•ca•no•ic acid

oc•ta•no•ic acid

OD
- optical density
- outside diameter

Oeh•ler
- O's symptom

Ogen

Ohm
- O's law

ohm

Oh•ni•shi
- Takayasu-O. disease

oil
- canola o.
- fish o.
- rapeseed o.

Ol•bert
- O. balloon catheter

old wom•an per•fo•ra•tion syn•drome

ole•ate

ole•ic acid

ole•in

ole•oyl

ol•i•go•car•dia

ol•i•gu•ria

Oli•ver
- O's sign

Om•ni•car•bon
- O. tilting-disk valve

Om•ni•paque

Om•ni•pen

Om•ni•science
- O. tilting-disk valve

On•co•vin

opac•i•ty
- vitreous o.

open•ing
aortic o.
aortic o. in diaphragm
atrioventricular o.
o. of coronary sinus
o. of inferior vena cava
o. of pulmonary trunk
o's of pulmonary veins
o. snap
o. of superior vena cava
o. for vena cava

op•er•a•tion (see also under *procedure*)
arterial switch o.
atrial switch o.
Blalock-Hanlon o.
Blalock-Hanlon atrial septectomy o.
Blalock-Taussig o.
Brock's o.
Fontan's o.
Glenn o.
Hunter's o.
Jatene o.
Matas' o.
Mustard o.
Potts o.
Rastelli's o.
Senning o.
Trendelenburg's o.
Vineberg o.
Waterston o.

oph•thal•mo•ple•gia
progressive external o.

oph•thal•mo•to•nom•e•try

opi•ate

Opitz
O. syndrome
O.-Frias syndrome
Smith-Lemli-O. syndrome

O point

Op•ti•ray

Ora•dex•on

Or•a•graf•in

Oram
Holt-O. syndrome

Ora•sone

Or•be•nin

Oret•ic

or•gan
o's of Zuckerkandl

or•i•fice
aortic o.
atrioventricular o.
auriculoventricular o.
o. of coronary sinus
o. of inferior vena cava
mitral o.
pulmonary o.
o. of pulmonary trunk
o. of superior vena cava
tricuspid o.

Or•ma•zine

orot•ic•ac•i•du•ria

Or•si
O.-Grocco method

or•tho•ar•te•ri•ot•o•ny

or•tho•per•cus•sion

or•tho•ples•sim•e•ter

or•thop•nea

or•tho•sta•sis

or•tho•stat•ic

or•tho•top•ic

Ort•ner
O's syndrome

OS
opening snap

Os
osmium

Os•borne
O. wave

os•cil•lo•gram

os•cil•lo•graph

os•cil•lom•e•ter

os•cil•lo•met•ric

os•cil•lom•e•try

os•cil•lo•scope

Os•ler
  O's disease
  O's nodes
  O's sign
  O's triad
  O.-Weber-Rendu disease
  Weber-O.-Rendu syndrome

Os•mi•trol

os•mi•um

Os•mo•glyn

os•mom•e•ter

os•si•fi•ca•tion
  pulmonary o.

os•teo•ar•thri•tis

os•teo•ar•throp•a•thy
  hypertrophic pulmonary o.

os•teo•gen•e•sis
  o. imperfecta (OI)

os•teo•gen•e•sis im•per•fec•ta syndrome, type I

os•teo•sar•co•ma
  extraskeletal o.

os•teo•tome

os•ti•um *pl.* os•tia
  o. aortae
  o. atrioventriculare dextrum
  o. atrioventriculare sinistrum
  coronary o.
  coronary sinus o.
  persistent o. primum
  o. secundum

os•ti•um *(continued)*
  o. sinus coronarii
  sinusoidal o.
  o. trunci pulmonalis
  o. venae cavae inferioris
  o. venae cavae superioris
  ostia venarum pulmonalium

Ost•wald
  O. viscosimeter

Osyp•ka
  O. lead
  O. screw-in lead

oua•ba•in

out•put
  cardiac o.
  left ventricular o.
  minute work o.
  pacemaker o.
  stroke o.
  stroke work o.
  work o. of the heart

over•drive

over•load
  diastolic o.
  pressure o.
  ventricular volume o.
  volume o.

over•load•ing
  pressure o.
  volume o.

over•sens•ing

over•sew•ing

over•shoot

ox•a•cil•lin so•di•um

ox•a•lo•sis

ox•an•dro•lone

ox•az•e•pam

ox•i•dase
  monoamine o.

ox•i•da•tion
beta o.
omega o.

ox•ide
mercuric o.
nitrous o.
intracardiac o.

Ox•i•met•rix
O. fiberoptic pulmonary artery catheter

ox•im•e•try
mixed venous o.

Ox-Pam

ox•pren•o•lol hy•dro•chlo•ride

Oxy•cel

ox•y•gen
o.-15

ox•y•ge•na•tion
extracorporeal membrane o. (ECMO)
gut mucosal o.
high-pressure o.
tissue o.

ox•y•ge•na•tor
bubble o.
extracorporeal membrane o.
membrane o.
pump-o.

oxy•phen•bu•ta•zone

oxy•ste•rol

P

P
phosphorus
programmable rate and/or output (pacemaker code)

P_{CO_2}
carbon dioxide partial pressure (tension)

P_{O_2}
oxygen partial pressure (tension)

PA
pulmonary artery

Pa
pulmonary arterial pressure

PAC
premature atrial contraction

pace•maker
AAI p.
AAIR p.
AAI-RR p.
AAT p.
activity-responsive p.
activity-sensing p.
antibradyarrhythmia p.
antitachycardia p.
AOO p.
artificial p.
ASVIP p.
asynchronous p.
asynchronous atrial p.
asynchronous electronic p.
asynchronous ventricular p.
atrial p.
atrial asynchronous p.
atrial demand p.
atrial demand inhibited p.
atrial demand inhibited–rate responsive p.

pace•maker *(continued)*
atrial demand triggered p.
atrial synchronous p.
atrial synchronous ventricular p.
atrial synchronous ventricular inhibited p.
atrioventricular asynchronous sequential p.
atrioventricular sequential p.
automatic p.
AV asynchronous sequential p.
AV junctional p.
AV sequential p.
AV universal p.
bipolar p.
cardiac p.
cardiac p., artificial
Chardack-Greatbatch p.
committed mode p.
Cyberlith p.
DDD p.
DDDR p.
DDI p.
demand p.
demand mode electronic p.
DOO p.
dual chamber p.
dual demand p.
DVI p.
ectopic p.
electronic p.
endocardial p.
epicardial p.
epicardial electronic p.
external p.
fixed p.
fixed-rate p.
fixed-rate electronic p.
fully automatic p.
p. of heart

pace•maker *(continued)*
implantable p.
implanted p.
internal p.
latent p.
p. lead
multiprogrammable p.
Nathan p.
permanent p.
p. pocket
programmable p.
prophylactic p.
P wave synchronous ventricular inhibited p.
QT-sensing p.
radio-frequency p.
rate-responsive p.
rechargeable p.
respiratory rate–dependent p.
runaway p.
secondary p.
shifting p.
single chamber p.
sinus p.
Spectrax programmable Medtronic p.
supraventricular p.
synchronous p.
synchronous electronic p.
temporary p.
temporary transvenous p.
transthoracic p.
transthoracic electronic p.
transvenous p.
two-timing p.
unipolar p.
universal p.
variable rate p.
VAT p.
VDD p.
ventricular p.
ventricular asynchronous p.
ventricular demand p.
ventricular demand inhibited p.

pace•maker *(continued)*
ventricular demand inhibited–rate responsive p.
ventricular demand triggered p.
ventricular inhibited electronic p.
VOO p.
VVI p.
VVIR p.
VVI-RR p.
VVT p.
wandering p.
wandering atrial p.

pace•maker syn•drome

pace•maker twid•dler's syn•drome

pace•map•ping

Pace•set•ter Syn•chro•ny

Pa•chon
P's test

pac•ing
AAI p.
AAT p.
AII p.
anodal p.
antitachycardia p.
AOO p.
asynchronous p.
asynchronous atrial p.
asynchronous ventricular p.
atrial p.
atrial fixed rate p.
atrial inhibited p.
atrial sequential p.
atrial synchronous p.
atrial synchronous ventricular p.
atrial triggered p.
atrioventricular asynchronous sequential p.

pac•ing *(continued)*
atrioventricular sequential p.
autodecremental p.
autodecremental overdrive p.
AV sequential p.
bifocal p.
bipolar p.
burst p.
cardiac p.
competitive p.
coupled atrial p.
coupled ventricular p.
DDD p.
DDI p.
demand p.
demand atrial p.
demand ventricular p.
dual chamber p.
dual demand p.
DVI p.
endocardial p.
epicardial p.
esophageal p.
fixed rate atrial p.
fixed rate ventricular p.
intracardiac p.
magnet p.
matched rate ventricular p.
noncompetitive ventricular p.
overdrive p.
paired p.
paired atrial p.
paired ventricular p.
patient-activated p.
permanent p.
physiologic p.
programmed p.
prophylactic p.
radiofrequency p.
rapid atrial p.
single chamber p.
tachycardia-reversion p.
temporary p.
p. threshold

pac•ing *(continued)*
transcutaneous p.
transmediastinal p.
transthoracic p.
transvenous p.
triggered atrial p.
triggered ventricular p.
underdrive p.
unipolar p.
VAT p.
VDD p.
ventricular p.
ventricular demand p.
ventricular fixed rate p.
ventricular inhibited p.
ventricular sequential p.
ventricular synchronous p.
ventricular triggered p.
VOO p.
VVI p.
VVT p.

pac•ing sys•tem
asynchronous p.s.
atrial triggered p.s.
automatic p.s.
demand p.s.
dual chamber fully automatic p.s.
inhibited p.s.
transvenous p.s.
triggered p.s.
universal p.s.

pack

pack-year

$PaCO_2$
arterial carbon dioxide pressure (tension)

$Paco_2$
arterial carbon dioxide pressure (tension)

PAD
peripheral arterial disease

pad
grounding p.

PAD (pulmonary artery diastolic) pres•sure

pad•dle
- defibrillator p's
- electrode p.
- external p's
- internal defibrillator p's

Pae•cilo•my•ces

PAEDP
- pulmonary artery end-diastolic pressure

Pa•get
- P. disease

pain
- abdominal p.
- chest p.
- musculoskeletal p.

pain•ful pace•maker pock•et syn•drome

P–A in•ter•val

Pa•lar•on

pal•la•di•um

Pal•lis•ter
- P.-Hall syndrome

pal•mi•tate

pal•mit•ic acid

pal•mi•tin

pal•mi•to•le•ate

pal•mi•to•le•ic acid

pal•mi•toyl

pal•mi•toyl•car•ni•tine

pal•mus

palp•a•ble

pal•pate

pal•pa•tion
- bimanual p.
- light touch p.

pal•pa•to•per•cus•sion

pal•pi•ta•tion

pal•sy
- ischemic p.

Pam•e•lor

PAN
- panarteritis nodosa

pan•an•gi•itis
- diffuse necrotizing p.

pan•ar•te•ri•tis
- p. nodosa

pan•car•di•tis

pan•cre•as *pl.* pan•cre•a•ta

pan•cre•a•ti•tis

pan•cu•ro•ni•um bro•mide

pan•cy•to•pe•nia
- congenital p.
- Fanconi's p.

pang
- breast p.

pan•my•elop•a•thy
- constitutional infantile p.

pan•nus

pan•sphyg•mo•graph

Pan•war•fin

pan•zer•herz

PaO_2
- arterial oxygen pressure (tension)

Pa_{O_2}
- arterial oxygen pressure (tension)

pa•pav•er•ine hy•dro•chlo•ride

para-ami•no•sal•i•cyl•ic acid

para-aor•tic

para•car•di•ac

para•cen•te•sis
  p. cordis
  p. pericardii
  p. thoracis

par•ac•et•a•mol

para•dox
  calcium p.
  oxygen p.

para•gan•gli•o•ma
  cardiac p.

para•gan•gli•on *pl.* para•gan•glia
  aortic p.
  cardiac p.

pa•ral•y•sis *pl.* pa•ral•y•ses
  ischemic p.
  periodic p.
  vasomotor p.
  Volkmann's ischemic p.

para•me•di•an

par•aor•tic

par•ar•rhyth•mia

para•ster•nal

para•sym•pa•thet•ic

para•sys•to•le
  atrial p.

para•ve•nous

Park
  P's aneurysm

Par•ker
  Bard-P. blade
  P. retractor

Par•kin•son
  Wolff-P.-White bypass tract
  Wolff-P.-White syndrome

Par•lo•del

Par•nate

par•ox•ys•mal

pars *pl.* par•tes
  p. abdominalis aortae
  p. ascendens aortae
  p. atlantica arteriae vertebralis
  p. atlantis arteriae vertebralis
  p. cavernosa arteriae carotidis internae
  p. cerebralis arteriae carotidis internae
  p. cervicalis arteriae carotidis internae
  p. cervicalis arteriae vertebralis
  p. descendens aortae
  p. infralobaris
  p. infrasegmentalis
  p. intersegmentalis
  p. intrasegmentalis
  p. membranacea septi atriorum
  p. membranacea septi interventricularis cordis
  p. muscularis septi interventricularis cordis
  p. petrosa arteriae carotidis internae
  p. prevertebralis arteriae vertebralis
  p. thoracica aortae
  p. transversa
  p. transversaria arteriae vertebralis
  p. umbilicalis

Par•son•net
  P. pouch

part
  sternocostal p. of diaphragm

par•tial tri•so•my 10q syn•drome

par•ti•cle
  VLDL remnant p's

par•ti•tion•ing
left atrial p.

pas•ser
right-angle p.
tie-on-p.

Pas•teur•el•la
P. multocida

PAT
paroxysmal atrial tachycardia

patch
Dacron p.
electrode p.
p. graft
MacCallum's p.
pericardial p.
plastic p.
prosthetic p.
soldiers' p's
Teflon p.
white p.
woven Dacron p.

patch•ing
transannular outflow tract p.

pat•en•cy
graft p.
probe p. of foramen ovale

pat•ent

Path•o•cil

path•way
accessory p.
accessory atrioventricular p.
accessory conducting p.
accessory conduction p.
anomalous p.
atrio-His p.
atrioventricular p.
AV conduction p.
cardiovascular reflex p.
circus p.
common collateral p's

path•way *(continued)*
concealed accessory p.
common p. of coagulation
extrinsic p. of coagulation
intrinsic p. of coagulation
macroreentrant p.
reentrant p.
retrograde p.
retrograde accessory conducting p.
scavenger cell p.
secondary p.

pa•tient-year

pat•tern
transmitral filling p.

pause
cardiac p.
compensatory p.
noncompensatory p.
post-extrasystolic p.
secondary p.
sinus p.
ventricular p.

Pa•va•bid

Pa•va•cap

Pav•a•cen

Pa•va•gen

Pa•va•rine

Pa•va•sed

Pa•va•tine

Pa•va•tym

Pa•ver•o•lan

Pav•u•lon

PAWP
pulmonary artery wedge pressure

Pb
lead (L. plumbum)

PBF
pulmonary blood flow

PCD
pacemaker/cardioverter/defibrillator

PCE Dis·per·tab

P cells

P_{CO_2}
carbon dioxide partial pressure (tension)

pCO_2
carbon dioxide partial pressure (tension)

$\mathit{p}CO_2$
carbon dioxide partial pressure (tension)

PCr
phosphocreatine

PCTA
percutaneous transluminal coronary angioplasty

PCWP
pulmonary capillary wedge pressure

Pd
palladium

PE
pulmonary embolism

Pé·an
P. clamp

pec·to·ral

pec·to·ra·lis

pec·tus *pl.* pec·to·ra
p. carinatum
p. excavatum

Pe·di·a·my·cin

PEEP
positive end-expiratory pressure

Pel·kan
Bloor, P., and Allen's method

pel·lag·ra

Pen·brit·in

pen·bu·to·lol sul·fate

pen·cil
electrocautery p.
electrosurgical p.

Pen·field
P. elevator

pen·i·cil·lin
benzathine p. G
p. G
p. G procaine
p. V

Pen·i·cil·li·um

pen·ta·eryth·ri·tol
p. tetranitrate

pen·tal·o·gy
p. of Fallot

pen·ta·mor·phone

pen·ta-X syn·drome

Pen·ta·zine

pen·taz·o·cine
p. hydrochloride
p. lactate

pen·to·bar·bi·tal
p. sodium

Pen·to·thal

pen·tox·i·fyl·line

Pen·tri·tol

Pen·ty·lan

PEP
preejection period

pep·tide
atrial natriuretic p. (ANP)
endocrine p.

pep•tide *(continued)*
neural p.

Pep•tol

per•cuss

per•cus•si•ble

per•cus•sion
auscultatory p.
bimanual p.
comparative p.
deep p.
direct p.
drop p.
drop stroke p.
finger p.
fist p.
Goldscheider's p.
immediate p.
instrumental p.
Korányi's p.
Lerch's p.
mediate p.
Murphy's p.
palpatory p.
pencil p.
piano p.
Plesch's p.
pleximetric p.
respiratory p.
slapping p.
strip p.
tangential p.
threshold p.
topographic p.

per•cus•sor

Pe•rez
P's sign

per•fo•ra•tion
cardiac p.
lead p.

per•for•mance
cardiac p.
left ventricular systolic p.
ventricular p.

per•fu•sion
continuous p.
coronary artery p.
myocardial p.
pulsatile p.

per•fu•sion•ist
pump p.

Per•heen•tu•pa
P. syndrome

peri•an•gi•itis

peri•aor•tic

peri•aor•ti•tis

peri•ar•te•ri•al

peri•ar•te•ri•tis
p. gummosa
p. nodosa
syphilitic p.

peri•atri•al

peri•au•ric•u•lar

peri•cap•il•lary

peri•car•dec•to•my

peri•car•di•ac

peri•car•di•al

peri•car•di•cen•te•sis

peri•car•di•ec•to•my

peri•car•dio•cen•te•sis

peri•car•di•ol•y•sis

peri•car•dio•me•di•as•ti•ni•tis

peri•car•dio•phren•ic

peri•car•dio•pleu•ral

peri•car•di•or•rha•phy

peri•car•di•os•to•my

peri•car•di•ot•o•my
limited p.
subxiphoid limited p.

peri•car•dit•ic

peri•car•di•tis
- acute p.
- acute benign p.
- acute fibrinous p.
- adhesive p.
- amebic p.
- bacterial p.
- calcific constrictive p.
- p. calculosa
- carcinomatous p.
- cholesterol p.
- chronic constrictive p.
- coccidioidomycosis p.
- constrictive p.
- drug-associated p.
- dry p.
- p. with effusion
- effusive constrictive p.
- elastic constrictive p.
- p. epistenocardiaca
- p. externa et interna
- external p.
- fibrinous p.
- fibrous p.
- fungal p.
- hemorrhagic p.
- histoplasmosis p.
- hypersensitivity-associated p.
- idiopathic p.
- infective p.
- localized p.
- mediastinal p.
- neoplastic p.
- p. obliterans
- obliterating p.
- parasitic p.
- postmyocardial infarction p.
- postoperative hemopericardium–associated p.
- purulent p.
- radiation p.
- recurrent p.
- rheumatic p.

peri•car•di•tis *(continued)*
- rheumatic fever–associated p.
- rheumatoid arthritis p.
- rigid constrictive p.
- scleroderma p.
- serofibrinous p.
- p. sicca
- suppurative p.
- systemic lupus erythematosus–associated p.
- toxin-associated p.
- traumatic p.
- tuberculous p.
- uremic p.
- p. villosa
- viral p.

peri•car•di•tis-myo•car•di•tis syn•drome

peri•car•di•um
- adherent p.
- bread-and-butter p.
- calcified p.
- cardiac p.
- p. fibrosum
- fibrous p.
- parietal p.
- p. serosum
- serous p.
- shaggy p.
- visceral p.

peri•car•dot•o•my

peri•cyte

peri•elec•trode

peri•graft

peri•myo•car•di•tis

peri•myo•en•do•car•di•tis

pe•ri•od
- absolute refractory p.
- effective refractory p.
- ejection p.
- p. of ejection

pe•ri•od *(continued)*
p. of filling
isoelectric p.
isometric p.
p. of isometric contraction
p. of isometric relaxation
isovolumetric p.
isovolumic p.
p. of isovolumic contraction
isovolumic relaxation p.
p. of isovolumic relaxation
mid-ejection p.
pacemaker refractory p.
postsphygmic p.
preejection p.
presphygmic p.
refractory p.
relative refractory p.
p. of slow ventricular filling
sphygmic p.
supernormal p.
systolic ejection p.
p. of ventricular filling
vulnerable p.
Wenckebach p.

pe•ri•o•dic•i•ty
circadian p.

peri•os•te•um

peri•phle•bit•ic

peri•phle•bi•tis
sclerosing p.

peri•por•tal

peri•py•le•phle•bi•tis

peri•the•li•al

peri•the•li•um

peri•tho•rac•ic

peri•to•neo•peri•car•di•al

peri•to•neo•peri•car•di•um

Per•i•trate

peri•val•vu•lar

peri•vas•cu•lar

peri•vas•cu•li•tis

peri•ve•nous

peri•ven•tric•u•lar

Per•ma-Hand suture

per•me•a•bil•i•ty
capillary p.

Per•san•tine

Per•thes
P. test

Per•to•frane

PES
programmed electrical stimulation

PET
positron emission tomography

pe•te•chia *pl.* pe•te•chiae

Pe•tit
P's sinus

PETN
pentaerythritol tetranitrate

Pe•tril•li•um

Pfi•zer•pen

PGE_2
prostaglandin E_2

PGI_2
prostacyclin

PH
pulmonary hypertension

pH
negative logarithm of hydrogen ion concentration

pHa
 arterial pH

phago•cy•to•sis

phar•ma•co•ki•net•ics

phar•ma•co•ther•a•py

phase
 p. 0
 p. 1
 p. 2
 p. 3
 p. 4
 atrial p.
 atrial contraction p.
 decreased ejection p.
 diastolic depolarization p.
 early rapid filling p.
 early rapid repolarization p.
 ejection p.
 filling p.
 final rapid repolarization p.
 isovolumetric p.
 isovolumetric contraction p.
 isovolumetric relaxation p.
 isovolumic p.
 isovolumic contraction p.
 isovolumic relaxation p.
 plateau p.
 rapid depolarization p.
 rapid ejection p.
 p. of rapid ejection
 rapid filling p.
 rapid inflow p.
 rapid ventricular filling p.
 p. of reduced ejection
 relaxation p.
 resting membrane potential p.
 slow filling p.
 slow ventricular filling p.
 upstroke p.
 ventricular filling p.
 ventricular isovolumic contraction p.

phase *(continued)*
 ventricular relaxation p.

Phe•na•meth

Phe•na•zine

Phen•cen

Phen•er•gan

phen•in•di•one

phe•no•bar•bi•tal
 p. sodium

Phe•no•ject

phe•nom•e•non *pl.* phe•nom•e•na
 Aschner's p.
 Ashman's p.
 Austin Flint p.
 Bowditch staircase p.
 Frank-Starling p.
 Gärtner's p.
 healing-over p.
 Litten's diaphragm p.
 Mobitz p.
 no-reflow p.
 Raynaud's p.
 R-on-T p.
 second-set p.
 staircase p.
 treppe p.
 warm-up p.
 Wenckebach p.

phe•no•per•i•dine

phe•no•thi•a•zine

phe•noxy•benz•amine hy•dro•chlo•ride

phen•tol•amine
 p. hydrochloride
 p. mesylate
 p. methanesulfonate

phen•yl•bu•ta•zone

phen•yl•eph•rine hy•dro•chlo•ride

phen•yl•pro•pa•nol•amine
p. hydrochloride
p. polistirex

phen•y•to•in
p. sodium

pheo•chro•mo•cy•to•ma

Phi•a•loph•o•ra

Phil•ips
P. gamma processor
P. whole-body 4-Tesla magnetic resonance system

PHLA
postheparin lipolytic activity

phleb•an•gi•o•ma

phleb•ar•te•ri•ec•ta•sia

phleb•as•the•nia

phleb•ec•ta•sia

phleb•ec•ta•sis

phleb•ec•to•my

phleb•ec•to•pia

phleb•ec•to•py

phleb•em•phrax•is

phleb•ex•air•e•sis

phle•bis•mus

phle•bit•ic

phle•bi•tis
adhesive p.
obliterating p.
obstructive p.
plastic p.
productive p.
proliferative p.
septic p.
suppurative p.

phlebo•fi•bro•sis

phle•bog•e•nous

phlebo•gram

phlebo•graph

phle•bog•ra•phy

phleb•oid

phlebo•lith

phlebo•li•thi•a•sis

phle•bol•o•gy

phlebo•ma•nom•e•ter

phlebo•phle•bos•to•my

phlebo•pi•ezom•e•try

phlebo•plas•ty

phlebo•rhe•og•ra•phy

phleb•or•rha•gia

phle•bor•rha•phy

phleb•or•rhex•is

phlebo•scle•ro•sis

phle•bo•sis

phleb•os•ta•sia

phle•bos•ta•sis

phlebo•ste•no•sis

phlebo•throm•bo•sis

phle•bot•o•my

phleg•ma•sia

pho•naco•scope

pho•na•cos•co•py

phon•ar•te•rio•gram

phon•ar•te•rio•graph•ic

phon•ar•te•ri•og•ra•phy

phon•en•do•scope

pho•no•an•gi•og•ra•phy

pho•no•aus•cul•ta•tion

pho•no•car•dio•gram

pho•no•car•dio•graph

pho•no•car•dio•graph•ic

pho•no•car•di•og•ra•phy
intracardiac p.

pho•no•cath•e•ter

pho•no•cath•e•ter•i•za•tion
intracardiac p.

pho•no•elec•tro•car•dio•scope

pho•no•gram

pho•no•scope

pho•nos•co•py

pho•no•stetho•graph

phos•phate
high-energy p.

phos•pha•ti•date

phos•pha•tide

phos•pha•ti•dic acid

phos•pha•ti•dyl•cho•line

phos•pha•ti•dyl•cho•line–ster•ol ac•yl•trans•fer•ase

phos•pha•ti•dyl•eth•a•nol•amine

phos•pho•cre•a•tine

phos•pho•di•es•ter•ase

6-phos•pho•fruc•to•ki•nase

phos•pho•hexo•isom•er•ase

phos•pho•lam•ban

phos•pho•lip•id

phos•pho•mono•es•ter•ase

phos•pho•rus

phos•phor•y•la•tion
oxidative p.

Phos•pho•tec

pho•to•cell
cadmium sulfide p.

pho•to•che•mo•ther•a•py

pho•to•de•tec•tor

pho•to•flu•o•rog•ra•phy

pho•to•hem•a•ta•chom•e•ter

pho•to•mi•cro•sur•gery

pho•ton

pho•to•peak

phreno•car•dia

phreno•peri•car•di•tis

pH-stat

phthal•im•i•dine

phthi•sis
aneurysmal p.

Phyl•lo•con•tin

phy•so•stig•mine

phy•to•ste•rol

Pick•er•ing
Lewis and P. test

pick•wick•i•an syn•drome

PICU
pediatric intensive care unit
pulmonary intensive care unit

PID (proportional plus integral plus derivative) feed•back

pi•esim•e•ter
Hales' p.

pi•ezo•car•dio•gram

pi•ezo•elec•tric

pi•ezo•elec•tric•i•ty

Pil•ling Wol•vek sternal approximator

pi•lo•car•pine

pin
    connector p.
    lead p.
    terminal p.

pin•do•lol

Pins
    P. sign

pi•per•a•cil•lin so•di•um

Pip•ra•cil

pir•bu•te•rol
    p. acetate
    p. hydrochloride

pi•re•tan•ide

Pi•ro•goff
    P's angle

pir•ox•i•mone

pix•el

plane
    cove p.
    frontal p.
    horizontal p.
    Ludwig's p.
    median p.
    sagittal p.
    sternoxiphoid p.
    subcostal p.
    suprasternal p.
    thoracic p.
    transpyloric p.
    umbilical p.

plaque
    atherosclerotic p.
    carcinoid p.
    fibrous p.
    Hollenhorst p's
    unstable p.

plas•ma
    fresh frozen p.

plas•ma•cy•to•ma

plas•ma•lem•ma

plas•ma•phe•re•sis
    serial exchange p.

plas•min

plas•min•o•gen

plate
    indifferent p.
    locking p.

pla•teau
    ventricular p.

plate•let
    blood p.

Pla•ti•nol

plat•i•num
    p.-iridium

pla•typ•nea

pled•get
    Teflon felt p.

Ple•gi•sol

Plesch
    P's percussion

ples•ses•the•sia

ples•si•graph

ple•thys•mo•gram

ple•thys•mo•graph
    digital p.
    finger p.

ple•thys•mog•ra•phy
    air-cuff p.
    dynamic venous p.
    impedance p.
    strain-gauge p.
    venous occlusion p.

pleu•ro•peri•car•di•al

pleu•ro•peri•car•di•tis

plex•im•e•ter

plex•i•met•ric

plex•im•e•try

plex•or

plex•us *pl.* plex•us, plex•us•es
- aortic p., abdominal
- aortic p., thoracic
- p. aorticus
- p. aorticus abdominalis
- p. aorticus thoracalis
- p. aorticus thoracicus
- areolar venous p.
- p. arteriae ovaricae
- Batson's p.
- cardiac p.
- cardiac p., anterior
- cardiac p., deep
- cardiac p., great
- cardiac p., superficial
- p. cardiacus
- p. cardiacus profundus
- p. cardiacus superficialis
- p. coronarius cordis anterior
- p. coronarius cordis posterior
- coronary p. of heart, anterior
- coronary p. of heart, left
- coronary p. of heart, posterior
- coronary p. of heart, right
- internal carotid venous p.
- perimuscular p.
- perimysial p.
- presacral p.
- prevertebral p's
- sacral p.
- sacral p., anterior
- p. sacralis anterior
- subendocardial terminal p.
- Trolard's p.
- vascular p.
- p. vasculosus
- p. venosus
- p. venosus canalis hypoglossi
- p. venosus caroticus internus
- p. venosus sacralis

plex•us *(continued)*
- p. venosus suboccipitalis
- p. venosus vertebralis externus anterior
- p. venosus vertebralis externus posterior
- p. venosus vertebralis internus anterior
- p. venosus vertebralis internus posterior
- venous p.
- venous p., sacral
- venous p., suboccipital
- venous p. of hypoglossal canal
- p. viscerales

pli•ca *pl.* pli•cae
- p. venae cavae sinistrae

plop
- tumor p.

plot
- bull's-eye p.
- polar p.

plu•to•ni•um

PMI
- point of maximal intensity

P-mi•trale

9p mono•so•my

PMS Ami•trip•ty•line

PMS Car•ba•ma•ze•pine

PMS Di•az•e•pam

PMS Flu•raz•e•pam

PMS Imip•ra•mine

PMS Iso•ni•a•zid

PMS Lor•a•ze•pam

PMS Me•tro•ni•da•zole

PMS Ox•az•e•pam

PMS Pro•meth•a•zine

PMS Pro•pran•o•lol

PMS Py•ra•zin•amide

PMS Sul•fa•sal•a•zine

PMS The•oph•yl•line

PMT
pacemaker-mediated tachycardia

PND
paroxysmal nocturnal dyspnea

pneu•ma•to•car•dia

pneu•mo•car•di•al

pneu•mo•car•dio•graph

pneu•mo•car•di•og•ra•phy

pneu•mo•he•mia

pneu•mo•he•mo•peri•car•di•um

pneu•mo•hy•dro•peri•car•di•um

pneu•mo•me•di•as•ti•num
acute spontaneous p.

pneu•mo•nia
eosinophilic p.

pneu•mo•ni•tis
hypersensitivity p.
rheumatic p.

pneu•mo•peri•car•di•um
tension p.

pneu•mo•pre•cor•di•um

pneu•mo•pyo•peri•car•di•um

pneu•mo•tacho•graph
Wolff integrating p.

pneu•mo•tho•rax
clicking p.

Po_2
oxygen partial pressure (tension)

pO_2
oxygen partial pressure (tension)

pO_2
oxygen partial pressure (tension)

pock•et
endocardial p's
dry p.
pacemaker p.
retroperitoneal p.
p's of Zahn

point
p. of Arrhigi
p. of critical stenosis
E p.
end-systolic p.
isoelectric p.
J p.
p. of maximal impulse
mitral valve E p.
O p.
pressure p.
pressure crossover p.

Poi•seuille
P. equation (Hagenbach extension)
P's space

po•lar•i•ty

po•lar•iza•tion
electrochemical p.

po•laro•graph•ic

Pol•he•mus
P.-Schafer-Ivemark syndrome

po•lio•my•eli•tis

poly•ac•rylo•ni•trile

poly•an•gi•itis

poly•ar•ter•itis
p. nodosa

Poly•cil•lin

Poly•cit•ra-K

poly•crot•ic

pol•yc•ro•tism

poly•cy•the•mia
  primary p. vera
  relative p. vera
  secondary p. vera
  p. vera

Poly•dek suture

poly•es•ter

poly•ether
  p. urethane

poly•eth•y•lene
  p. glycol
  p. terephthalate

poly•glac•tin
  p. 370
  p. 910

poly•gly•col•ic acid

poly•graph

Poly•mox

poly•my•al•gia rheu•ma•ti•ca syn•drome

poly•myo•si•tis

pol•yp
  cardiac p.

poly•pro•py•lene

poly•sple•nia syn•drome

poly•sty•rene
  sodium p. sulfonate

poly•thi•a•zide

poly•un•sat•u•rat•ed

poly•ure•thane
  segmented p.

poly•vi•nyl
  p. pyridine
  p. chloride

poly•vi•nyl•pyr•rol•i•done
  p.-iodine

Pom•pe
  P's disease

pool
  blood p.

por•phy•ria
  acute intermittent p.

por•ta•ca•val

Por•ter
  P's sign

por•to•sys•tem•ic

po•si•tion•ing
  Gantry p.

pos•i•tron

POST
  posterior

post•ax•i•al ac•ro•fa•cial dys•os•to•sis syn•drome

post•cap•il•lary

post•car•di•ot•o•my

post•ca•va

post•ca•val

post•di•as•tol•ic

post•di•crot•ic

pos•te•ri•ad

pos•te•ri•or

pos•tero•an•te•ri•or

pos•tero•ex•ter•nal

pos•tero•in•fe•ri•or

pos•tero•in•ter•nal

pos•tero•lat•er•al

pos•tero•me•di•al

pos•tero•me•di•an

pos•tero•su•pe•ri•or

post•ex•tra•sys•tol•ic

post•im•plan•ta•tion

post•in•farct

post-op
postoperative

post•per•fu•sion

post•peri•car•di•ot•o•my

post•peri•car•di•ot•o•my syn•drome

post•sphyg•mic

post•ste•not•ic

post•trans•plan•ta•tion

Po•tain
P's sign

po•tas•si•um
p. acetate
p. bicarbonate
p. canrenoate
p. chloride
p. citrate
p. glucaldrate
p. gluconate
glucose-insulin-p.
p. hydroxide
p. phosphate

po•ten•tial
action p.
after-p.
bioelectric p.
cardiac resting p.
depressed fast-response action p.
diastolic p.
electrochemical p.
fast-response action p.
intracardiac p.
maximal diastolic p.
membrane p.
musculoskeletal p.
pacemaker p.
resting p.
resting membrane p.

po•ten•tial *(continued)*
slow-response action p.
threshold p.
transmembrane p.

po•ten•ti•a•tion
post-extrasystolic p.
p. by radiation

po•ten•ti•om•e•ter

Pott
P's aneurysm

Potts
P. ductus clamp
P. operation
P. procedure
P. scissors
P. shunt

pouch
Parsonnet p.

po•vi•done
p.-iodine

pow•er
left ventricular p.
nonelastic p.

pow•er cell
alpha-emitting nuclear p.c.
BCX p.c.
beta-voltaic p.c.
biogalvanic hybrid fuel p.c.
bromine complex (BCX) p.c.
Celsa p.c.
double anode p.c.
double-barrier wrap p.c.
electrochemical p.c.
external p.c.
gamma-emitting nuclear p.c.
lithium anode p.c.
lithium-bromine p.c.
lithium–copper sulfide p.c.
lithium-iodine p.c.
lithium-iodine double anode p.c.

pow•er cell *(continued)*
lithium–lead iodide p.c.
lithium–lead sulfide p.c.
lithium–manganese dioxide p.c.
lithium–silver chromate p.c.
lithium–thionyl chloride p.c.
lithium–titanium disulfide p.c.
mercury p.c.
mercury-zinc p.c.
nickel-cadmium p.c.
nuclear p.c.
plutonium p.c.
polyvinyl pyridine p.c.
promethium p.c.
rechargeable p.c.
Ruben Mallory p.c.
SAFT p.c.
silver-mercury–silver-zinc p.c.
thermoelectric p.c.
zinc-mercury p.c.

PPH
primary pulmonary hypertension

P–P in•ter•val

P-pul•mo•nale

PQ in•ter•val

prac•to•lol

pra•va•sta•tin
p. sodium

pra•zo•sin hy•dro•chlo•ride

pre•aor•tic

pre•be•ta-lipo•pro•tein
sinking p.

pre•cap•il•lary

pre•car•di•ac

pre•car•di•um

pre•ca•va

pre•clot

pre•clot•ting

pre•cor•dia

pre•cor•di•al

pre•cor•di•al•gia

pre•cor•di•um

pre•di•as•to•le

pre•di•a•stol•ic

pre•di•crot•ic

Pred•ni•cen-M

pred•nis•o•lone
p. acetate
p. hemisuccinate
p. sodium phosphate
p. sodium succinate
p. steaglate
p. tebutate

pred•ni•sone

pre•eclamp•sia

pre•ejec•tion

pre•ero•sion

pre•ex•ci•ta•tion
ventricular p.

pre•im•plan•ta•tion

pre•kal•li•kre•in
A-mode p.

pre-β-lipo•pro•tein
sinking p.

pre•load
ventricular p.

Pre•lone

Prem•a•rin

pre•ma•ture cor•o•nary ar•te•ry dis•ease

pre•med•i•ca•tion

pre•nal•ter•ol
p. hydrochloride

pre-op
preoperative (before surgery)

pre•pon•der•ance
ventricular p.

pre•po•ten•tial

pres•by•car•dia

pre•scle•rot•ic

pre•sen•ta•tion
B-mode p.
M-mode p.

pres•er•va•tion
perfusion p.

pre•sphyg•mic

pres•som•e•ter

pres•sure
aortic p.
arterial p.
back p.
blood p.
capillary p.
cardiac transmural distending p.
carotid p.
central venous p. (CVP)
continuous positive airway p. (CPAP)
coronary perfusion p.
critical closing p.
diastolic p.
diastolic filling p.
endocardial p.
high blood p.
intra-abdominal p.
intra-arterial p.
intracardiac p.
intrapericardial p.
intrathoracic p.
intravascular p.
intraventricular p.
jugular venous p.

pres•sure *(continued)*
left atrial p.
left atrial mean p.
left ventricular p.
left ventricular diastolic p.
left ventricular end-diastolic p.
left ventricular filling p.
mean arterial p.
mean circulatory filling p.
oncotic p.
operating diastolic p.
PAD p.
paradoxical blood p.
perfusion p.
plasma colloid osmotic p.
positive end-expiratory p. (PEEP)
pullback p.
pulmonary arterial p.
pulmonary artery p.
pulmonary artery diastolic p.
pulmonary artery end-diastolic p.
pulmonary artery occlusion p.
pulmonary artery occlusive wedge p.
pulmonary artery wedge p.
pulmonary capillary p.
pulmonary capillary wedge p.
pulmonary venous p.
pulse p.
resting p.
right atrial p.
right atrial mean p.
right ventricular p.
right ventricular systolic p.
systolic p.
venous p.
ventricular diastolic p.
ventricular filling p.
wedged hepatic vein p.

pre•sys•to•le

pre•sys•tol•ic

pre-β-VLDL
very-low-density lipoprotein

Pri•max•in

Prin•ci•pen

prin•ci•ple
Fick p.
Frank-Starling p.

Prin•i•vil

Prin•zide

Prinz•me•tal
P's angina pectoris

Pris•co•line

Pro-50

pro•ar•rhyth•mic

Pro-Ban•thine

probe
biplane p.
bipolar pacing p.
blood flow p.
nonimaging nuclear p.
nuclear p.
pacing p.
pediatric p.
scintillation p.
transluminal pacing p.

pro•bu•col

pro•cain•amide hy•dro•chlo•ride

Pro•can

Pro•car•dia

pro•ce•dure (see also under *operation*)
direct Fick p.
endocardial resection p.
extended endocardial resection p.
Fick p.

pro•ce•dure *(continued)*
Fontan p.
Glenn p.
invasive p.
Konno p.
Mustard atrial switch p.
noninvasive p.
Potts p.
Rashkind p.
right ventricular disconnection p.
Senning p.
Senning atrial switch p.

pro•ces•sor
Philips gamma p.

pro•co•ag•u•lant

Pro•cy•tox

pro•dro•mal

prod•uct
fibrin split p.
fibrinogen degradation p.
fibrinogen-fibrin degradation p.
pressure rate p.
rate-pressure p.

pro•fun•da•plas•ty

Pro•gens

pro•ge•ria

Pro•gly•cem

prog•no•sis

prog•nos•ti•ca•tion

pro•gram
Honolulu Heart P.
Hypertension Detection and Follow-up P.
National Cholesterol Education P.
New England Regional Infant Cardiac P.
Vario p.

pro•gram•ma•bil•i•ty

pro•gram•mer
Cordis Omnicor p.
CPI p.
magnetic field p.
Medtronic p.
Pacesetter p.
universal p.

pro•gram•ming
phantom p.
radiofrequency p.
ultrasonic p.

proj•ect
Coronary Drug P.
Pooling P.

pro•jec•tion
LAO p's

pro•lapse
mitral p.
mitral valve p.

Pro•lene

Pro•lene suture

pro•lon•ga•tion
AH interval p.
drug-induced QT interval p.
HV interval p.
PR interval p.
QT interval p.

Pro•lo•prim

Pro•meth

pro•meth•a•zine hy•dro•chlo•ride

pro•me•thi•um
p. 147

Pro•mine

Pro•nes•tyl

pro•pa•fen•one
p. hydrochloride

pro•pan•the•line bro•mide

pro•pel•lant
halogenated hydrocarbon p.

pro•phy•lac•tic

pro•phy•lax•is
early rejection p.

pro•po•fol

pro•pran•o•lol
p. hydrochloride
p. LA

pro•pyl•bu•tyl•do•pa•mine

pro•pyl•ene
p. carbonate

pro•pyl•thio•ura•cil

Pro•pyl-Thy•ra•cil

pros•ta•cy•clin

pros•ta•glan•din
PGE_1
PGE_2
PGI_2

pros•ta•noid

Pro•staph•lin

pros•the•sis *pl.* pros•the•ses
aortic p.
Beall valve p.
Beall-Surgitool valve p.
bifurcated vessel p.
Björk-Shiley valve p.
Braunwald-Cutter valve p.
caged-ball p.
cardiac valve p.
Carpentier-Edwards valve p.
Cooley-Cutter valve p.
Cross-Jones valve p.
DeBakey-Surgitool valve p.
Duromedics p.
Hall-Kaster valve p.
Hancock porcine valve p.
Hancock valve p.

pros•the•sis *(continued)*
Harken valve p.
heart valve p.
Ionescu-Shiley valve p.
Kay-Shiley valve p.
Kay-Suzuki valve p.
knitted vascular p.
Lillehei-Kaster pivoting-disk valve p.
Magovern-Cromie valve p.
Meadox-Gabbay valve p.
mechanical p.
Medtronic-Hall valve p.
mitral p.
Omnicarbon tilting-disk valve p.
Omniscience tilting-disk valve p.
pivoting-disk valve p.
porcine valve p.
Smeloff-Cutter valve p.
St. Jude Medical valve p.
Starr-Edwards valve p.
Surgitool valve p.
tilting-disk p.
vascular p.
Wada-Cutter valve p.

pro•ta•mine
p. sulfate

pro•tec•tion
hypothermic p.
myocardial p.

pro•tec•tor
wound p.

pro•tein
C p.
p. C
coagulation p.
contractile p.
M line p.
p. S

pro•tein ki•nase A

pro•tein ki•nase C

pro•tein•o•sis
alveolar p.

Pro•tha•zine

pro•throm•bin

pro•throm•bin•ase

pro•to•col
Balke p.
Balke-Ware p.
Bruce p.
Bruce treadmill p.
Ellestad p.
modified Bruce p.
Naughton p.
Naughton treadmill p.
Scandanavian p.
treadmill exercise test p.
treadmill stress testing p.
triangular p.

pro•to•di•a•stol•ic

Pro•to•stat

Pro•trin

pro•trip•ty•line hy•dro•chlo•ride

pro-uro•ki•nase

Pro•ven•til

Pro•vo•cho•line

Pro•zac

PRQ
pressure-rate quotient

P–R seg•ment

PRU
peripheral resistance unit

pseud•an•gi•na

pseu•do•an•eu•rysm

pseu•do•an•gi•na

pseu•do•cap•sule

pseu•do•cho•lin•es•ter•ase

pseu•do•clau•di•ca•tion

pseu•do•co•arc•ta•tion
    p. of the aorta

pseu•do•cur•rent
    p. of injury

pseu•do•dex•tro•car•dia

pseu•do•di•a•stol•ic

pseu•do•fu•sion

pseu•do•he•mo•phil•ia

pseu•do-Hur•ler poly•dys•tro•phy syndrome

pseu•do•hy•po•ten•sion

pseu•do•in•farc•tion

pseu•do•mal•func•tion

Pseu•do•mo•nas
    P. aeruginosa

pseu•do•peri•car•di•al

pseu•do•tha•lid•o•mide syn•drome

pseu•do•thrill

pseu•do•trun•cus ar•te•ri•o•sus

pseu•do•valve

pseu•do•xan•tho•ma elas•ti•cum

psit•ta•co•sis

pso•ri•a•sis

PSS
    progressive systemic sclerosis

PSVT
    paroxysmal supraventricular tachycardia

psy•cho•stim•u•lant

$4p^-$ syndrome

$5p^-$ syndrome

$9p^-$ syndrome

Pt
    platinum

PTCA
    percutaneous transluminal coronary angioplasty

Pu
    plutonium

puff

pul•mo•aor•tic

Pul•mo•lite

pul•mo•nale
    pseudo-P p.

pul•mo•nary

pul•mon•ic

Pul•moph•yl•line

pul•sa•tile

pul•sa•tion
    cardiac p.
    expansile p.
    suprasternal p.

pulse
    abdominal p.
    abrupt p.
    allorhythmic p.
    alternating p.
    p. amplitude
    anacrotic p.
    anadicrotic p.
    anatricrotic p.
    apical p.
    arterial p.
    atrial liver p.
    atrial venous p.
    atriovenous p.
    biferious p.
    bigeminal p.
    bisferiens p.
    bisferious p.
    cannon ball p.
    capillary p.

pulse *(continued)*
carotid p.
catadicrotic p.
catatricrotic p.
centripetal venous p.
collapsing p.
Corrigan's p.
coupled p.
dicrotic p.
digitalate p.
dropped-beat p.
elastic p.
epigastric p.
equal p.
febrile p.
filiform p.
formicant p.
frequent p.
full p.
hard p.
high-tension p.
infrequent p.
intermittent p.
irregular p.
jerky p.
jugular p.
jugular venous p.
Kussmaul's p.
labile p.
low-tension p.
missing p.
Monneret's p.
monocrotic p.
nail p.
pacemaker output p.
pacing p.
paradoxical p.
parvus et tardus p.
pedal p.
pistol-shot p.
plateau p.
polycrotic p.
quadrigeminal p.
quick p.
Quincke's p.
radial p.
respiratory p.
retrosternal p.

pulse *(continued)*
Riegel's p.
running p.
sharp p.
short p.
slow p.
soft p.
strong p.
tense p.
thready p.
tricrotic p.
trigeminal p.
trip-hammer p.
undulating p.
unequal p.
vagus p.
venous p.
vermicular p.
vibrating p.
water-hammer p.
wiry p.

pulse gen•er•a•tor
AAI p.g.
AAT p.g.
abdominal p.g.
asynchronous p.g.
biological p.g.
bipolar p.g.
constant voltage p.g.
Cordis p.g.
CPI p.g.
explanted p.g.
external p.g.
implantable p.g.
Interlith p.g.
Medtronic Xyrel p.g.
multiprogammable p.g.
runaway p.g.
synchronous p.g.
unipolar p.g.
Vario voltage threshold–measuring p.g.
VVI p.g.
VVT p.g.
zinc-mercury p.g.

pulse•less dis•ease

pul•sus *pl.* pul•sus
- p. abdominalis
- p. aequalis
- p. alternans
- p. biferiens
- p. bigeminus
- p. bisferiens
- p. celer
- p. differens
- p. filiformis
- p. formicans
- p. fortis
- p. frequens
- p. irregularis perpetuus
- p. magnus
- p. magnus et celer
- p. mollis
- p. monocrotus
- p. oppressus
- p. paradoxus
- p. parvus
- p. parvus et tardus
- p. plenus
- p. tardus
- p. trigeminus
- p. undulosus
- p. vacuus
- p. venosus

pump
- arterial p.
- balloon p.
- booster p.
- calcium p.
- cardiac balloon p.
- centrifugal p.
- heart-lung p.
- heparin-coated pulsatile p.
- heparin-coated roller p.
- Impeller p.
- intra-aortic balloon p.
- Na^+-K^+ p.
- percutaneous intra-aortic balloon p.
- pulsatile p.
- roller p.
- sodium p.
- sodium-potassium p.

pump-oxy•gen•a•tor

punch
- aortic p.
- biopsy p.
- Karp aortic p.
- sternal p.
- Sweet sternal p.

punc•ture
- arterial p.
- direct apical left ventricular p.
- femoral vein p.
- left ventricular p.
- percutaneous p.
- subclavian p.

pu•pil
- Argyll Robertson p.
- Robertson's p.

Pur•kin•je
- His-P. conduction time
- His-P. system
- P. bridge
- P's cells
- P. fibers
- P. layer
- P. network
- P. system
- terminal conducting fibers of P.

pur•pu•ra
- allergic p.
- anaphylactoid p.
- fibrinolytic p.
- p. fibrinolytica
- p. fulminans
- p. hemorrhagica
- Henoch's p.
- Henoch-Schönlein p.
- idiopathic p.
- p. nervosa
- nonthrombocytopenic p.
- p. rheumatica
- Schönlein p.
- Schönlein-Henoch p.
- thrombocytopenic p.

pur•pu•ra *(continued)*
  thrombocytopenic p., idiopathic
  thrombocytopenic p., secondary
  thrombocytopenic p., thrombotic
  thrombopenic p.

pur•pu•ric

PVB
  premature ventricular beat

PVC
  polyvinyl chloride
  premature ventricular contraction

PVR
  pulmonary vascular resistance

P wave

PW (pulsed wave) Dop•pler imag•ing

py•elo•ne•phri•tis
  chronic p.
  unilateral p.

py•e•mia
  arterial p.
  portal p.

py•le•phle•bec•ta•sis

py•le•phle•bi•tis
  adhesive p.

py•le•throm•bo•phle•bi•tis

py•le•throm•bo•sis

py•lic

Pyo•pen

pyo•peri•car•di•tis

pyo•peri•car•di•um

pyo•pneu•mo•peri•car•di•um

PYP
  pyrophosphate

py•ra•zin•amide

pyr•i•dine
  polyvinyl p.

Py•ro•lite

py•ro•phos•phate
  stannous p.

py•ru•vate

py•ru•vic acid

Q

Q fever

QRS al·ter·nans

QRS com·plex

QRS in·ter·val

QRST in·ter·val

QS com·plex

13q$^-$ syndrome

18q$^-$ syndrome

Q–Tc in·ter·val

Q–T in·ter·val

quad·ri·cus·pid

quad·ri·gem·i·ny

Quain
    Q's fatty heart

Quel·i·cin

Qué·nu
    Q.-Muret sign

Ques·tran

Ques·tran Light

Quet·e·let
    Q. index

Qui·bron-T

Quick
    Q. tourniquet test

Quincke
    Q's pulse
    Q's sign

quin·eth·a·zone

quin·i·dine
    q. gluconate
    q. sulfate

qui·nine
    q. sulfate

quo·tient
    pressure-rate q.

Q wave

R

R
  rate modulation (pacemaker code)
  resistance
  roentgen

R
  resistance

Ra
  radium

rab•bit
  Watanabe heritable hyperlipidemic (WHHL) r.

RAD
  right axis deviation

rad
  absorbed dose of ionizing radiation

ra•dar•ky•mog•ra•phy

ra•di•al apla•sia–throm•bo•cy•to•pe•nia syn•drome

ra•di•a•tion
  potentiation by r.

rad•i•cal
  free r.
  hydroxyl r.
  oxygen r.
  peroxide r.
  superoxide r.

ra•dic•u•li•tis
  cervical r.

ra•dio•ac•tiv•i•ty

ra•dio•car•dio•gram

ra•dio•car•di•og•ra•phy

ra•dio•elec•tro•car•dio•gram

ra•dio•elec•tro•car•di•o•graph

ra•dio•elec•tro•car•di•og•ra•phy

ra•dio•graph

ra•dio•graph•ic

ra•di•og•ra•phy
  chest r.

ra•dio•im•mu•no•as•say

ra•dio•ky•mog•ra•phy

ra•dio•la•bel

ra•di•ol•o•gist

ra•di•ol•o•gy

ra•dio•lu•cen•cy

ra•dio•lu•cent

ra•dio•nu•clide

ra•dio-opac•i•ty

ra•di•opac•i•ty

ra•di•opaque

ra•dio•par•en•cy

ra•dio•par•ent

ra•dio•phar•ma•ceu•ti•cal
  single-photon r.

ra•dio•tra•cer

ra•dio•trans•par•en•cy

ra•dio•trans•par•ent

ra•di•um

ra•dix *pl.* ra•di•ces
  radices parietales venae cavae inferioris
  radices viscerales venae cavae inferioris

ra•don

RAE
  right atrial enlargement

rale
pulmonary r.

ra•mus *pl.* ra•mi
r. acetabularis arteriae circumflexae femoris medialis
r. acetabularis arteriae obturatoriae
r. acetabuli arteriae circumflexae femoris medialis
r. acromialis arteriae suprascapularis
r. acromialis arteriae thoraco-acromialis
r. acromialis arteriae transversae scapulae
r. anterior arteriae obturatoriae
r. anterior arteriae pancreaticoduodenalis inferioris
r. anterior arteriae recurrentis ulnaris
r. anterior arteriae renalis
r. anterior arteriae thyroideae superioris
rami arteriosi interlobulares hepatis
rami articulares arteriae descendentis genicularis
rami articulares arteriae genus descendentis
r. ascendens arteriae circumflexae femoris lateralis
r. ascendens arteriae circumflexae femoris medialis
r. ascendens arteriae circumflexae ilium profundae
r. ascendens arteriae transversae colli
r. ascendens rami superficialis arteriae transversae cervicis

ra•mus *(continued)*
r. atrialis anastomoticus arteriae coronariae sinistrae
rami atriales arteriae coronariae dextrae
rami atriales arteriae coronariae sinistrae
r. atrialis intermedius arteriae coronariae dextrae
r. atrialis intermedius rami circumflexi arteriae coronariae sinistri
rami atrioventriculares arteriae coronariae sinistrae
rami bronchiales arteriae mammariae internae
rami cardiaci cervicales inferiores nervi vagi
rami cardiaci cervicales superiores nervi vagi
rami cardiaci inferiores nervi recurrentis
rami cardiaci thoracici nervi vagi
rami caroticotympanici arteriae carotidis internae
rami caudati
r. circumflexus arteriae coronariae sinistrae
r. circumflexus fibulae arteriae tibialis posterioris
r. circumflexus fibularis arteriae tibialis posterioris
r. clavicularis arteriae thoracoacromialis
r. collateralis arteriarum intercostalium posteriorum
r. communicans
r. communicans arteriae fibularis

ra•mus *(continued)*
- r. communicans arteriae peroneae
- r. coni arteriosi arteriae coronariae dextrae
- r. coni arteriosi arteriae coronariae sinistrae
- r. costalis lateralis arteriae mammariae internae
- r. costalis lateralis arteriae thoracicae internae
- r. cutaneus lateralis arteriarum intercostalium posteriorum
- r. cutaneus lateralis rami dorsalis arteriarum intercostalium posteriorum
- r. cutaneus medialis rami dorsalis arteriarum intercostalium posteriorum
- r. deltoideus arteriae profundae brachii
- r. deltoideus arteriae thoracoacromialis
- r. descendens anterior arteriae coronariae [cordis] sinistrae
- r. descendens arteriae circumflexae femoris lateralis
- r. descendens posterior arteriae coronariae [cordis] dextrae
- r. descendens rami superficialis arteriae transversae cervicis
- r. dexter arteriae hepaticae propriae
- r. dexter arteriae pulmonalis
- r. dexter venae portae hepatis

ra•mus *(continued)*
- r. dorsalis arteriarum intercostalium posteriorum
- rami dorsales arteriae intercostalis supremae
- r. dorsalis arteriarum lumbalium
- r. dorsalis arteriae subcostalis
- r. dorsalis venarum intercostalium
- r. dorsalis venarum intercostalium posteriorum [IV–XI]
- rami esophagei aortae thoracicae
- rami esophagei arteriae gastricae sinistrae
- rami esophagei arteriae thyroideae inferioris
- r. glandularis anterior arteriae thyreoideae superioris
- rami glandulares arteriae thyreoideae inferioris
- rami glandulares arteriae thyreoideae superioris
- r. glandularis lateralis arteriae thyreoideae superioris
- r. glandularis posterior arteriae thyreoideae superioris
- r. hyoideus arteriae lingualis
- r. hyoideus arteriae thyreoideae superioris
- r. iliacus arteriae iliolumbalis
- r. inferior arteriae gluteae superioris
- r. infrahyoideus arteriae thyroideae superioris
- rami inguinales arteriae femoralis
- rami intercostales anteriores arteriae thoracicae internae

ra•mus *(continued)*
rami intercostales arteriae mammariae internae
r. interventricularis anterior arteriae coronariae sinistrae
r. interventricularis posterior arteriae coronariae dextrae
rami interventriculares septales
r. lateralis interventricularis anterioris arteriae coronariae sinistrae
r. lumbalis arteriae iliolumbalis
rami mammarii
r. marginalis dexter
r. marginalis sinister
rami mediastinales aortae thoracalis
rami mediastinales aortae thoracicae
rami mediastinales arteriae thoracicae internae
rami musculares arteriae vertebralis
r. nodi atrioventricularis arteriae coronariae dextrae
r. nodi atrioventricularis arteriae coronariae sinistrae
r. nodi sinuatrialis arteriae coronariae dextrae
r. nodi sinuatrialis arteriae coronariae sinistrae
rami oesophagei aortae thoracicae
rami oesophagei arteriae gastricae sinistrae
rami oesophagei arteriae thyroideae inferioris
rami pancreatici

ra•mus *(continued)*
rami parietales aortae abdominalis
rami parietales aortae thoracalis
rami parietales arteriae hypogastricae
rami pectorales arteriae thoracoacromialis
r. perforans arteriae fibularis
rami perforantes arteriae mammariae internae
r. perforans arteriae peroneae
rami perforantes arteriae thoracicae internae
rami pericardiaci aortae thoracalis
rami pericardiaci aortae thoracicae
r. posterior arteriae obturatoriae
r. posterior arteriae recurrentis ulnaris
r. posterior arteriae renalis
r. posterior arteriae thyroideae superioris
r. posterior ventriculi sinistri
r. posterolateralis dexter
r. profundus arteriae circumflexae femoris medialis
r. profundus arteriae gluteae superioris
r. profundus arteriae transversae cervicis
r. profundus arteriae transversae colli
rami radiculares arteriae vertebralis
rami sacrales laterales arteriae sacralis medianae

ra•mus *(continued)*
r. saphenus arteriae descendentis genicularis
r. saphenus arteriae genus descendentis
r. sinister arteriae hepaticae propriae
r. sinister arteriae pulmonalis
r. sinister venae portae hepatis
rami spinales arteriae cervicalis ascendentis
r. spinalis arteriae iliolumbalis
rami spinales arteriae intercostalis supremae
r. spinalis arteriarum lumbalium
rami spinales arteriarum sacralium lateralium
r. spinalis arteriae subcostalis
rami spinales arteriae vertebralis
r. spinalis rami dorsalis arteriarum intercostalium posteriorum
r. spinalis rami lumbalis arteriae iliolumbalis
r. spinalis venarum intercostalium
r. spinalis venarum intercostalium posteriorum [IV–XI]
rami splenici arteriae splenicae
rami sternales arteriae mammariae internae
rami sternales arteriae thoracicae internae
rami sternocleidomastoidei arteriae occipitalis
rami subendocardiales
rami subscapulares arteriae axillaris

ra•mus *(continued)*
r. superficialis arteriae circumflexae femoris medialis
r. superficialis arteriae gluteae superioris
r. superficialis arteriae transversae cervicis
r. superficialis arteriae transversae colli
r. superior arteriae gluteae superioris
rami thymici arteriae thoracicae internae
r. transversus arteriae circumflexae femoris lateralis
r. transversus arteriae circumflexae femoris medialis
r. ventriculi sinistri posterior
rami viscerales aortae abdominalis
rami viscerales aortae thoracalis
rami viscerales arteriae hypogastricae

ran•cid

RAO
right anterior oblique

RAP
right atrial pressure

Rash•kind
R. balloon septostomy
R's procedure

Ras•mus•sen
R's aneurysm

ras•pa•to•ry
Alexander rib r.
Doyen rib r.
Haight rib r.
rib r.

Ras•tel•li
R's operation
R. repair
R. technique

rate
circulation r.
compliance r.
count r.
disintegration r.
r. drift
erythrocyte sedimentation r. (ESR)
escape r.
heart r.
impulse formation r.
intrinsic myocardial washout r.
net myocardial washout r.
pacing r.
oxidation r.
peak diastolic filling r.
pulse r.
resting heart r.
sinus node impulse formation r.
slew r.
target heart r.

rat•ing
r. of perceived exertion

ra•tio
AV conduction r.
cardiothoracic r.
conduction r.
ventilation-perfusion r.

Rau•ber
hepatic funiculus of R.

Rau•wol•fia
R. serpentina

ray
beta r's
gamma r's
x-r's

Ray•naud
R's disease

Ray•naud *(continued)*
R's gangrene
R's phenomenon
R's sign

Rb
rubidium

RBB
right bundle branch

RBBB
right bundle branch block

RCA
right coronary artery

RC (resistance-capacitance) cir•cuit

re•ac•tion
alarm r.
allograft r.
digitonin r.
Fenton r.
fibrinolytic r.
fight-or-flight r.
Haber-Weiss r.
homograft r.
inflammatory r.
Liebermann-Burchard r.
pyrogen r.
second-set r.

re•a•gin

re•anas•to•mose

re•an•as•to•mo•sis

re•can•al•iza•tion

re•can•nu•la•tion

re•cep•tor
chylomicron remnant r.
LDL r.
low-density lipoprotein (LDL) r's
muscarinic r's

re•cess
aorticomediastinal r.

re•cip•i•ent
organ transplant r.

Reck•ling•haus•en
R's tonometer

re•cord•ing
biplane r.
Doppler r.
His bundle r.
M-mode r.
MAP r.
pull-back r.
transtelephonic ECG r.

rec•ti•fi•ca•tion
anomalous r.
inward-going r.

re•duc•tion
afterload r.

re•dun•dant cusp syn•drome

re•en•try
anatomical r.
atrial r.
atrioventricular nodal r.
AV nodal r.
functional r.
sinus r.
ventricular r.

re•fill
transcapillary r.

re•flec•tion
pericardial r.

re•flex
accelerator r.
aortic r.
Aschner's r.
atriopressor r.
Bainbridge r.
baroreceptor r.
Bezold r.
Bezold-Jarisch r.
cardiac r.
cardiac depressor r.
cardiac respiratory r.
carotidosympathoatrial r.

re•flex *(continued)*
carotidovagoatrial r.
carotidoventricular r.
carotid sinus r.
chemoreceptor r.
coronary r.
deep tendon r. (DTR)
eyeball compression r.
eyeball-heart r.
intercoronary r.
ischemic r.
oculocardiac r.
oculovagal r.
pericardial r.
pressor r.
pressoreceptor r.
psychocardiac r.
pulmonocoronary r.
vascular r.
vasopressor r's
vasovagal r.
viscerocardiac r.

re•flux
abdominojugular r.
esophageal r.
hepatojugular r.

re•frac•tor•i•ness
postrepolarization r.

re•gion
AN r.
H r.
infarct r.
N r.
NH r.
noninfarct r.
precordial r.

reg•is•try
ablation r.
angioplasty r.
CASS r.
Coronary Artery Surgery Study r.
National Heart, Lung, and Blood Institute R.
NHLBI R.
valvuloplasty r.

Reg•i•tine

reg•u•la•tion
α-stat r.
pH-stat r.

re•gur•gi•ta•tion
acute mitral r.
aortic r.
aortic valve r.
luetic aortic r.
mitral r.
mitral valve r.
nonrheumatic mitral r.
normal valvular r.
pulmonary r.
pulmonic r.
pulmonic valvular r.
semilunar valve r.
tricuspid r.
valvular r.

re•ha•bil•i•ta•tion
cardiac r.
in-hospital cardiac r.
vocational r.
work r.

Reil
band of R.

re•in•farc•tion

re•in•fu•sion
in-line r.

re•in•ner•va•tion

Rei•ter
R's disease
R's syndrome

re•jec•tion
acute r.
acute cellular r.
allograft r.
bad beat r.
cardiac allograft r.
cardiac transplant r.
cellular r.
chronic r.
first-set r.

re•jec•tion *(continued)*
graft r.
hyperacute r.
second-set r.
transplant r.

re•la•tion
diastolic pressure-volume r.
end-diastolic pressure-volume r.
end-systolic pressure-volume r.
end-systolic stress-dimension r.
force-frequency r.
force-length r.
force-velocity r.
force-velocity-length r.
Frank-Starling r.
length–resting tension r.
length-tension r.
pressure-volume r.
Starling r.
ventilation-perfusion r.
ventricular end-systolic pressure-volume r.

re•la•tion•ship
length-tension r.

re•lax•ant
muscle r.

re•lax•a•tion
cardiac muscle r.
isovolumetric r.
isovolumic r.
stress r.
ventricular r.

re•lease
aortic cross-clamp r.
cross-clamp r.

rem

Re•mak
R's ganglion

rem•nant
chylomicron r's

re•mod•eling

Ren•du
  Osler-Weber-R. disease
  Weber-Osler-R. syndrome

Ren•ese

re•nin

re•nin•o•ma

Re•no•graf•in

Reno-M

Reno-M-Dip

re•no•vas•cu•lar

Re•no•vist

re•op•er•a•tion

re•ox•y•gen•a•tion

re•pair
  Fontan r.
  Rastelli r.

re•per•fu•sion
  myocardial r.

re•place•ment
  crystalloid volume r.
  valve r.

re•po•lar•iza•tion
  atrial r.
  early r.
  ventricular r.

Rep-Pred

re•pres•sion

re•pro•gram•ming
  inadvertent r.
  spurious r.

re•sect

re•sec•tion
  endocardial r.
  heart wall r.
  myotomy-myectomy-septal r.
  septal r.

Re•serf•ia

res•er•pine

re•serve
  cardiac r.
  coronary arterial r.
  coronary flow r.
  diastolic r.
  extraction r.
  heart rate r.
  left ventricular r.
  preload r.
  systolic r.
  vasodilator r.

re•ser•voir
  venous r.

res•in
  anion exchange r.
  bile acid–binding r.
  cholestyramine r.
  epoxy r.
  ion exchange r.
  sequestrant r.

re•sis•tance
  airway r.
  coronary vascular r.
  peripheral r.
  pulmonary vascular r.
  systemic vascular r.
  total peripheral r.
  vascular r.
  vascular peripheral r.

res•o•lu•tion
  contrast r.
  energy r.
  spatial r.
  temporal r.
  vector r.

res•o•nance
  cine magnetic r.
  electron paramagnetic r. (EPR)
  magnetic r.
  nuclear magnetic r.
  tympanic r.

res•o•nance *(continued)*
vesicular r.
vesiculotympanic r.

res•o•nant

re•sor•ci•nol•phthal•e•in

Resp•bid

res•pi•ra•tion
Cheyne-Stokes r.
mouth-to-mouth r.

res•pi•rom•e•ter
Kofranyi-Michaelis r.

re•sponse
Cushing pressure r.
frequency r.
giving-up–given-up r.
immune r.

rest
embryonic r.

re•ste•no•sis
false r.
true r.

re•sus•ci•ta•tion
cardiac r.
cardiopulmonary r. (CPR)
r. of the heart

re•sus•ci•ta•tor
cardiopulmonary r.

re•te *pl.* re•tia
acromial r.
r. acromiale
r. arteriosum
articular r.
articular cubital r.
articular r. of knee
r. articulare cubiti
r. articulare genus
r. canalis hypoglossi
r. olecrani
r. of patella
r. patellae
r. patellare
r. vasculosum articulare

re•te *(continued)*
r. venosum
retia venosa vertebrarum

re•ten•tion
fluid r.
sodium r.
water r.

re•tic•u•lum *pl.* re•tic•u•la
Chiari's r.
sarcoplasmic r.

ret•i•nop•a•thy

re•trac•tor
Allison lung r.
atrial r.
Beckman self-retaining r.
Carpentier combined sternal-atrial r.
Cooley r.
Cooley atrial r.
Crile r.
Davidson scapular r.
Deaver r.
Finochietto r.
flat ribbon r.
Gelpi r.
Goulet r.
Harrington r.
Israel r.
Langenbeck r.
lung r.
malleable r.
Murphy r.
Parker r.
rake r.
Richardson r.
Sauerbruch r.
scapular r.
self-retaining r.
Senn r.
sternal r.
US Army r.
vein r.
Volkman r.
Weinberg r.
Weitlaner r.

re•trans•fu•sion

ret•ro•esoph•a•ge•al

ret•ro•grade

ret•ro•ster•nal

re•turn
venous r.

Ret•zi•us
R. veins

re•vas•cu•lar•iza•tion
coronary r.
myocardial r.

Re•ver•sol

re•view
Cineloop digital image r.

Re•vi•mine

re•warm•ing

RF
regurgitant fraction
rheumatic fever

RFW
rapid filling wave

Rh
rhodium

rhab•do•my•o•ma
cardiac r.

rhab•do•myo•sar•co•ma
cardiac r.

rhe•ol•o•gy

rho•di•um

Rho•tri•mine

rhythm
2:1 r.
accelerated r.
accelerated idiojunctional r.
accelerated idioventricular r.
accelerated junctional r.

rhythm *(continued)*
accelerated nodal r.
atrial r.
atrioventricular r.
atrioventricular junctional r.
automatic r.
AV junctional r.
AV sequential electronic pacemaker r.
baseline r.
cantering r.
cardiac r.
circadian r.
coupled r.
r. of development
delta r.
ectopic r.
escape r.
r. of excitation
gallop r.
idiojunctional r.
idionodal r.
idioventricular r.
junctional r.
junctional escape r.
nodal r.
nodal accelerated r.
normal sinus r.
pacing r.
pendulum r.
quadruple r.
reciprocal r.
reciprocating r.
sinoatrial r.
sinus r.
r. strip
triple r.
ventricular r.
ventricular accelerated r.

rhyth•mic•i•ty

RIA
radioimmunoassay

rib
r. approximator
r. contractor

rib *(continued)*
- r. raspatory
- r. shears

Rib•bert
- R's thrombosis

ri•bo•nu•cle•ase

ri•bose

Rich
- Hamman-R. syndrome

Rich•ard•son
- R. retractor

Ri•chet
- R's aneurysm

ri•cin•ole•ic acid

RID
- radial immunodiffusion

Rie•gel
- R's pulse

rif•am•pin

rig•or
- calcium r.

Ri•ley
- R.-Day syndrome

Rind•fleisch
- R's folds

ring
- r. of aorta
- aortic r.
- aortic valve r.
- atrioventricular r.
- atrioventricular valve r.
- Carpentier r.
- Carpentier tricuspid r.
- Crawford suture r.
- fibrous r's of heart
- Lower's r's
- mitral r.
- mitral valve r.
- prosthetic valve sewing r.
- pulmonary r.
- pulmonary valve r.

ring *(continued)*
- sewing r.
- suture r.
- tricuspid r.
- tricuspid valve r.
- valve r.
- vascular r.
- r. of Vieussens

Rit•a•lin

Ri•ve•ro
- R.-Carvallo sign

RKY
- roentgenkymography

RLAT
- right lateral

RMP
- resting membrane potential

RMS Uni•serts

Rn
- radon

RNase
- ribonuclease

Rob•ert
- Simpson-R. catheter

Rob•erts-SC pho•co•me•lia syn•drome

Rob•ert•son
- R's pupil

Robi•my•cin

Ro•bi•now
- R's dwarfism
- R's syndrome

Rob•in•son
- French-R. catheter
- R's circle

Ro•bi•nul

Rod•ri•gues
- R. aneurysm

roent•gen

roent•gen•ky•mo•graph

roent•gen•ky•mog•ra•phy

roent•geno•car•dio•gram

roent•geno•gram
chest r.

roent•geno•graph

roent•geno•graph•ic

roent•gen•og•ra•phy
cardiac r.
chest r.

roent•geno•ky•mo•graph

Ro•ger
bruit de R.
maladie de R.
R's bruit
R's disease
R's murmur

Ro•gers
R. needle holder

ro•gor

roll•er
Davis r.

Ro•ma•ña
R's sign

Ro•ma•no
R.-Ward syndrome

Ro-My•cin

ron•geur

R-on-T phe•nom•e•non

root
r. of aorta
aortic r.

Ro•sen•bach
R's syndrome

Ros•tan
R's asthma

Rotch
R's sign

Roth
R's spots

Roth•ia
R. dentocariosa

Rou•bac

Roug•non
R.-Heberden disease

Rous•sy
R-Lévy disease
R-Lévy hereditary areflexic dystasia
R.-Lévy syndrome

Rox•an•ol

RPA
right pulmonary artery

RPE
rating of perceived exertion

RPP
rate-pressure product

RR (cardiac cycle length) in•ter•val

rTPA
recombinant tissue plasminogen activator

rt-PA
recombinant tissue plasminogen activator

rub
friction r.
pericardial r.
pericardial friction r.

rub•ber
silicone r.

ru•bel•la

Ru•ben Mal•lory battery

Ru•ben Mal•lory power cell

ru•be•o•la

Ru•bex

ru•bid•i•um
- r.-81
- r.-82
- r. chloride Rb 86
- r. Rb 82

Ru•bin•stein
- R's syndrome
- R.-Taybi syndrome

rule
- Simpson's r.

rum•ble
- mid-diastolic r.
- mid-diastolic flow r.

Ru•mel
- R. thoracic forceps
- R. tourniquet

rup•ture
- r. of aorta
- cardiac r.
- myocardial r.
- nonpenetrating cardiac r.
- penetrating cardiac r.

Rus•sian forceps

Ru•val•ca•ba
- R's syndrome

RV
- right ventricle

RVEF
- right ventricular ejection fraction

RVG
- radionuclide ventriculography

RVH
- right ventricular hypertrophy

RVSWI
- right ventricular stroke work index

R wave

Ryth•mo•dan

Ryth•mol

S

S
- shock (pacemaker code)
- single chamber (pacemaker code)
- sulfur

SA
- sinoatrial
- sinus arrest

S-A
- sinoatrial

S-AB
- sinoatrial block

sac
- aneurysmal s.
- heart s.
- pericardial s.
- ventral aortic s.

Sac•cha•ro•my•ces

Sacks
- Libman-S. disease
- Libman-S. endocarditis
- Libman-S. syndrome

Sae•thre
- S.-Chotzen syndrome

St. Vi•tus
- St. V. dance

Sa•ka•ki•ba•ra
- Konno-S. bioptome

Sal•a•zo•py•rin

sal•a•zo•sul•fa•pyr•i•dine

sal•bu•ta•mol

sal•i•cyl•ate

Sal•kow•ski
- S's test

Sal•mo•nel•la

sal•mo•nel•la *pl.* sal•mo•nel•lae

salt
- chromic s's

Sal•u•ron

sal•vage
- blood s.
- continuous cell s.
- myocardial s.

SAM
- systolic anterior motion

Sand•im•mune

san•guif•er•ous

san•gui•mo•tor

san•gui•mo•to•ry

SA (sinoatrial) node

San•sert

San•som
- S's sign

SAP
- systolic arterial pressure

sa•phe•na

sa•pon•i•fi•ca•tion

Sap•pey
- veins of S.

sar•coi•do•sis
- s. cordis

sar•co•lem•ma

sar•co•ma *pl.* sar•co•mas, sar•co•ma•ta
- Kaposi's s.
- neurogenic cardiac s.
- synovial cardiac s.

sar•co•mere

Sarns
- S. electric saw
- S. vent

Sar•ot
S. bronchus clamp

S.A.S.

Sa•tin•sky
S. vascular clamp

sat•u•rat•ed

sat•u•ra•tion
arterial oxygen s. (SaO_2)
mixed venous oxygen s.
oxygen s.

Sau•er•bruch
S. retractor
S. rib shears

sav•er
Haemonetics Cell S.

saw
electric s.
Sarns electric s.
sternal s.

Sayre
Kearns-S. syndrome

Sb
antimony (L. stibium)

SBF
systemic blood flow

SBP
systolic arterial blood pressure

scale
Borg s.
French s.

sca•le•nus an•ti•cus syn•drome

scal•pel

scan
CAT s.
cine CT s.
CT s.
first pass s.
gated s.

scan *(continued)*
magnetic resonance imaging (MRI) s.
M-mode s.
MUGA (multiple gated acquisition) s.
real time s.
scintillation s.
ultrasound s.

scan•ner
cine computed tomography s.
cine CT s.
CT s.
fast computed tomography s.
fast CT s.
millisecond CT s.

scan•ning
blood pool s.
computed tomography s.
CT s.
gated cardiac blood pool s.
gated CT s.
infarct avid s.
MUGA s.
multiple gated acquisition s.
perfusion exercise s.
perfusion lung s.
radionuclide s.
technetium Tc-99m pyrophosphate s.
thallium-201 s.
thallium-201 exercise s.
ventilation-perfusion lung s.

scat•ter
Compton s.

Scha•fer
Polhemus-S.-Ivemark syndrome

Scheie
Hurler-S. compound

Scheie *(continued)*
Hurler-S. compound syndrome
S's syndrome

Schiff
S's test

Schin•zel
S.-Giedion syndrome

schis•to•so•mi•a•sis

Schnei•der
S's indicator

Schnidt
S. clamp

Schön•lein
Henoch-S. purpura
Henoch-S. syndrome
S's disease
S. purpura
S.-Henoch purpura
S.-Henoch syndrome

scin•ti•gram
pyrophosphate s.

scin•ti•graph

scin•tig•ra•phy
acute infarct s.
acute myocardial infarction s.
Anger camera s.
cardiac s.
dipyridamole thallium-201 s.
exercise myocardial perfusion s.
exercise thallium s.
first pass s.
gated cardiac blood pool s.
infarct avid s.
infarct avid myocardial s.
myocardial s.
myocardial infarction s.
myocardial perfusion s.
perfusion s.

scin•tig•ra•phy *(continued)*
pulmonary s.
pulmonary perfusion s.
PYP s.
pyrophosphate s.
resting thallium s.
stress s.
stress myocardial perfusion s.
stress thallium s.
Tc-99m pyrophosphate s.
technetium Tc-99m pyrophosphate s.
technetium Tc-99m stannous pyrophosphate s.
thallium stress s.
thallium-201 s.
thallium-201 myocardial perfusion s.
thallium-201 perfusion s.
ventilation s.
ventricular function s.

scin•til•la•tion cam•era
multicrystal s.c.
single crystal s.c.

scin•ti•scan

scis•sors
cardiovascular s.
curved s.
curved Mayo s.
DeMartel s.
Diethrich coronary s.
Diethrich valve s.
dissecting s.
Litwak mitral valve s.
Mayo s.
Metzenbaum s.
Nelson s.
Potts s.
right angle s.
vascular s.

scle•ra *pl.* scle•rae
blue s.

scle•ro•der•ma

scle•ro•gen•ic

scle•rog•e•nous

scle•ros•ing

scle•ro•sis
  accelerated coronary s.
  aortic s.
  arterial s.
  arteriocapillary s.
  arteriolar s.
  endocardial s.
  hyperplastic s.
  medial calcific s.
  Mönckeberg's s.
  progressive systemic s.
  subendocardial s.
  tuberous s.
  valvular s.
  vascular s.
  venous s.

scle•rot•ic

sco•pol•a•mine
  s. butylbromide
  s. hydrobromide

score
  jeopardy s.
  Killip clinical s.
  treadmill exercise s.
  wall motion s.

screen•ing
  antibody s.
  lymphocytotoxic antibody s.

screw
  endomyocardial s.
  set s.
  three-turn epicardial s.

scu-PA
  single chain urokinase-type plasminogen activator

scur•vy

Se
  selenium

seal
  crimp s.
  hermetic s.

seal•ing
  crimp s.

Sec•tral

seg•ment
  coved ST s.
  PQ s.
  P–R s.
  ST s.
  Ta s.
  T–P–Q s.

Sel•din•ger
  S. technique

se•le•ni•um

self-dis•charge

self-test•ing

Senn
  S. retractor

Sen•ning
  S. interatrial baffle
  S. operation
  S. procedure

sens•ing
  all-or-none s.
  atrial s.
  ventricular s.

sen•sor
  polarographic oxygen s.

SEP
  systolic ejection period

sep•a•ra•tion
  E point–septal s.

SE (Starr-Edwards) prosthetic valve

sep•sis
  gram-negative s.

sep•tal

sep•tec•to•my
atrial s.
Blalock-Hanlon atrial s.

sep•ti•ce•mia

sep•to•mar•gi•nal

sep•tos•to•my
balloon s.
balloon atrial s.
Rashkind balloon s.

sep•tot•o•my
balloon atrial s.

Sep•tra

sep•tum *pl.* sep•ta
atrial s.
atrioventricular s. of heart
s. atrioventriculare cordis
bulbar s.
interatrial s. of heart
s. interatriale cordis
interauricular s.
interventricular s. of heart
s. interventriculare cordis
parietal s.
perimembranous s.
s. primum
s. secundum
s. of ventricles of heart
ventricular s.
s. ventriculorum cordis

se•quence
bilateral left-sidedness s.
bilateral right-sidedness s.
DiGeorge s.
laterality s.
linear sebaceous nevus s.
pulse s.
spin-echo imaging s.
Sturge-Weber s.

se•ques•trant
bile acid s.

se•ques•tra•tion

Ser•ax

Ser•ial•Vue system

sero•to•nin

Ser•pa•lan

Ser•pa•sil

Ser•ra•tia

se•rum *pl.* se•rums, se•ra
pericardial s.

se•rum glu•ta•mic-ox•a•lo•ace•tic trans•am•i•nase (SGOT)

se•rum glu•ta•mic-ox•a•lo•ace•tic trans•fer•ase (SGOT)

set
coronary artery s.
Diethrich coronary artery bypass instrument s.

Se•ven Coun•tries Study

SFW
slow filling wave

S_3 gal•lop

S_4 gal•lop

SGOT
serum glutamic-oxaloacetic transaminase
serum glutamic-oxaloacetic transferase

shad•ow
heart s.

Sharp
Brown and S. gauge

Shaw
S. monitoring system

shears
- Bethune rib s.
- Gluck rib s.
- rib s.
- Sauerbruch rib s.
- Shoemaker rib s.
- Stille-Giertz rib s.

Shee•han
- S. and Dodge method

shell
- ejection s.

Shi•ley
- Björk-S. convexoconcave prosthetic valve
- Björk-S. monostrut prosthetic valve
- Björk-S. prosthetic valve
- Ionescu-S. pericardial valve
- Ionescu-S. prosthetic valve

shock
- cardiac s.
- cardiogenic s.
- declamping s.
- diastolic s.
- distributive s.
- hematogenic s.
- hemorrhagic s.
- hypovolemic s.
- irreversible s.
- obstructive s.
- oligemic s.
- regional s.
- secondary s.
- septic s.
- synchronized s.
- toxic s.
- vasogenic s.
- warm s.

Shoe•mak•er
- S. rib shears

shor•ten•ing
- fractional myocardial s.
- ventricular wall s.

short PR syn•drome

Shprin•tzen
- S's syndrome

shud•der
- carotid s.

Shultze
- S's test

shunt
- aortopulmonary s.
- arteriovenous (A-V) s.
- bidirectional s.
- Blalock s.
- Blalock-Taussig s.
- cardiac s.
- cardiovascular s.
- Glenn s.
- Gore-Tex s.
- Gott s.
- internal s.
- intracardiac s.
- Javid s.
- left-to-right s.
- portacaval s.
- postcaval s.
- Potts s.
- reversed s.
- right-to-left s.
- subclavian pulmonary s.
- systemic pulmonary s.
- unidirectional s.
- Vitagraft arteriovenous s.
- Waterston s.

Shy
- S.-Drager syndrome

Si
- silicon

Sib•son
- S's notch
- S's vestibule

sick•le cell dis•ease

sick•ness
- African sleeping s.

sick•ness *(continued)*
mountain s.

sid•ed•ness
cardiac s.

sid•er•o•sis
myocardial s.

SIDS
sudden infant death syndrome

Sie•mens
S.-Elema lead connector
S.-Elema pacemaker lead
S.-Elema ribbon lead

Sie•mens Cor•os•kop C single plane angiocardiography system

sign
Aschner's s.
Auenbrugger's s.
auscultatory s.
Bamberger's s.
Bouillaud's s.
Bozzolo's s.
Branham's s.
Braunwald s.
Brickner's s.
Broadbent's s.
Broadbent's inverted s.
Brockenbrough's s.
calcium s.
Cardarelli's s.
Carvallo s.
Castellino's s.
Cegka's s.
Corrigan's s.
Delbet's s.
de Musset's s.
Dorendorf's s.
Drummond's s.
Duchenne's s.
Duroziez's s.
Ebstein's s.
epicardial fat pad s.
Ewart's s.
Fischer's s.

sign *(continued)*
Friedreich's s.
Glasgow's s.
Gowers' s.
Gunn's crossing s.
Hall's s.
Hamman's s.
Heim-Kreysig s.
Hill's s.
Homans' s.
Hope's s.
Jaccoud's s.
knuckle s.
Kreysig's s.
Kussmaul's s.
Levine's s.
Litten's s.
McGinn-White s.
Mahler's s.
Moschcowitz's s.
Müller's s.
Musset's s.
Nicoladoni's s.
Nicoladoni-Branham s.
Oliver's s.
Osler's s.
Perez's s.
Pins' s.
Porter's s.
Potain's s.
Quénu-Muret s.
Quincke's s.
Raynaud's s.
Rivero-Carvallo s.
Romaña's s.
Rotch's s.
Sansom's s.
square root s.
Traube's s.
vein s.
Westermark's s.

sig•nal
Doppler s.

Si•las•tic

sil•hou•ette
cardiac s.

sil•hou•ette *(continued)*
cardiopericardial s.
cardiovascular s.

sil•i•con
s. germanium

sil•i•cone
s. rubber

silk
braided s.

sil•ver
s. chromate

Simp•son
S. atherectomy catheter
S's rule
S's rule formula
S.-Robert catheter

sim•u•la•tor
electrocardiographic s.

sim•vas•ta•tin

Sin•e•quan

sin•is•tro•car•dia

si•no•atri•al

si•no•atri•al syn•drome

si•no•au•ric•u•lar

si•no•gram

si•no•spi•ral

sinu•at•ri•al

si•nus *pl.* si•nus, si•nus•es
s. aortae
s. aortae [Valsalvae]
aortic s.
s. arteriae pulmonalis
s. caroticus
carotid s.
s. coronarius
coronary s.
s. of internal jugular vein, inferior
s. of internal jugular vein, superior

si•nus *(continued)*
s. of Morgagni
oblique s. of pericardium
s. obliquus pericardii
s. pericardii
Petit's s.
posteustachian s.
s's of pulmonary trunk
s. of spleen
splenic s.
s. splenicus
transverse s. of pericardium
s. transversus pericardii
s. trunci pulmonalis
s. of Valsalva
s. of venae cavae
s. venarum cavarum
s. venosus
venous s.

si•nu•soid

si•nu•spi•ral

si•nus syn•drome

site
aortic entry s.

β-si•tos•ter•ol

β-si•tos•ter•ol•emia

si•tus *pl.* si•tus
s. inversus
s. inversus totalis
s. inversus viscerum
s. perversus
s. solitus
s. transversus

siz•er
prosthetic valve s.

SK
streptokinase

skel•e•ton
cardiac s.
fibrous s. of heart
s. of heart

skin
  plastic s.
  velour s. button

SK-Pra•mine

sleeve
  protective s.
  silicone rubber anchor s.

Slo-Bid

Slo-Ni•a•cin

Slo-Phyl•lin

Slow-Tra•si•cor

sludg•ing

Sly
  S's syndrome

Smith
  S.-Lemli-Opitz syndrome

smok•ing
  cigarette s.

Smyth code

Sn
  tin (L. stannum)

snap
  mitral opening s.
  opening s.
  tricuspid opening s.

SNP
  sodium nitroprusside

So•ci•e•ty for Car•di•ac An•gi•og•ra•phy

So•ci•e•ty of Car•dio•vas•cu•lar An•es•the•si•ol•o•gists

So•ci•e•ty for Vas•cu•lar Sur•gery

SOD
  superoxide dismutase

so•di•um
  aspirin, s. bicarbonate, and citric acid
  s. bicarbonate
  dietary s.
  s. hydroxide
  s. nitrite
  s. nitroprusside
  s. pertechnetate Tc 99m
  s. polystyrene sulfonate
  vascular s.

Soem•mer•ing
  arterial veins of S.
  external radial vein of S.

So•far•in

Sol•fo•ton

Solu-Cor•tef

Solu-Med•rol

Solu-Phyl•lin

Sol•u•rex

so•lu•tion
  bacitracin s.
  bacitracin-saline s.
  cardioplegic s.
  fixative s.
  heparin and normal saline s.
  heparinized physiological s.
  heparinized saline s.
  ice-cold physiological s.
  normal saline s.
  physiological s.
  saline s.

so•ma•to•stat•in

Som•no•thane

So•mo•phyl•lin

Som-Pam

Sones
  S. coronary angiography
  S. coronary arteriography

Sones *(continued)*
S. coronary arteriography catheter
S. coronary catheter
S. technique

So•no•clot analysis

Sor•bi•trate

so•roche

So•ta•cor

so•ta•lol hy•dro•chlo•ride

souf•fle
cardiac s.
continuous mammary s.
mammary s.
systolic mammary s.

sound
aortic ejection s.
aortic second s.
atrial s.
auscultatory s.
bellows s.
cardiac s's
ejection s's
extracardiac s.
first s.
first heart s.
flapping s.
fourth s.
fourth heart s.
friction s.
heart s's
Korotkoff s's
nonejection systolic s.
pacemaker s.
percussion s.
pericardial s.
pericardial friction s.
pistol-shot s.
prosthetic valve s.
pulmonic ejection s.
pulmonic second s.
S_1 s.
S_2 s.
S_3 s.

sound *(continued)*
S_4 s.
sail s.
second s.
second heart s.
S_3 gallop s.
S_4 gallop s.
single second heart s.
summation s.
systolic ejection s's
third s.
third heart s.
tick-tack s's
to-and-fro s.
valvular ejection s.
vascular ejection s.
water-wheel s.

space
H. s.
Holzknecht's s.
intercostal s.
intravascular s.
Poiseuille's s.
prevertebral s.
retrocardiac s.
Traube's s.
Westberg's s.

Span-Ni•a•cin

spasm
arterial s.
catheter-induced s.
coronary s.
coronary artery s.
esophageal s.

SPECT
single-photon emission computed tomography

spec•tros•co•py
magnetic resonance s.
proton s.

spec•trum *pl.* spec•tra
facio-auriculo-vertebral s.

spell
  hypoxic s.

Spens
  S. syndrome

sphinc·ter
  hepatic s.
  precapillary s.

sphin·go·lip·i·do·sis

sphin·go·my·e·lin

sphyg·mic

sphyg·mo·car·dio·gram

sphyg·mo·car·dio·graph

sphyg·mo·car·dio·scope

sphyg·mo·chro·no·graph

sphyg·mo·dy·na·mom·e·ter

sphyg·mo·gram

sphyg·mo·graph

sphyg·mo·graph·ic

sphyg·mog·ra·phy

sphyg·moid

sphyg·mol·o·gy

sphyg·mo·ma·nom·e·ter
  aneroid s.

sphyg·mom·e·ter

sphyg·mo·met·ro·graph

sphyg·mo·met·ro·scope

sphyg·mo-os·cil·lom·e·ter

sphyg·mo·pal·pa·tion

sphyg·mo·phone

sphyg·mo·ple·thys·mo·graph

sphyg·mo·scope
  Bishop's s.

sphyg·mos·co·py

sphyg·mo·sys·to·le

sphyg·mo·to·nom·e·ter

sphyg·mo·vis·co·sim·e·try

spike
  marker s.

spill·over
  norepinephrine s.

spin·dle
  aortic s.
  His' s.

spir·o·no·lac·tone

sple·no·meg·a·ly
  congestive s.
  thrombophlebitic s.

split·ting
  broad fixed s. of S_2
  fixed s. of S_2
  s. of heart sounds
  paradoxical s. of S_2
  reversed s.
  reversed s. of S_2
  wide s. of S_2

spon·dy·li·tis
  ankylosing s.

spon·dy·lo·ar·throp·a·thy

sponge
  4 × 4 s.
  absorbable s.
  absorbable gelatin s.
  dissecting s.
  s. dissector
  s. forceps
  four by four s.
  gauze s.
  gelatin s.
  lap s.
  laparotomy s.
  s. stick

spot
  Brushfield's s's
  cold s.
  hot s.
  milk s's

spot *(continued)*
Roth's s's
soldier's s's

spu•tum

squal•ene

squat•ting

Sr
strontium

SSS
sick sinus syndrome

ST
sinus tachycardia

stand
cardiovascular imaging s.
Mayo s.

stand•ing

stand•still
atrial s.
auricular s.
cardiac s.
sinus s.
ventricular s.

Stan•ford
S. bioptome

Stan•ley Kent
bundle of S.K.

Staph•cil•lin

Staph•y•lo•coc•cus
S. aureus
S. epidermidis

staph•y•lo•coc•cus *pl.* staph•y•lo•coc•ci

sta•ple
skin s.

starch
hydroxyethyl s.

Star•ling
Frank-S. curve
Frank-S. effect

Star•ling *(continued)*
Frank-S. law
Frank-S. mechanism of the heart
Frank-S. phenomenon
Frank-S. principle
Frank-S. relation
S. curve
S. equation
S. forces
S's law of the heart
S. mechanism
S. relation

Starr
S.-Edwards caged-ball valve
S.-Edwards prosthetic valve

sta•sis
pressure s.
venous s.

state
basal s.
high cardiac output s.
hypercoagulable s.
inotropic s.
low output s.
polarized s.
primary hypercoagulable s.
resting s.
secondary hypercoagulable s.

Sta•tex

Stat•i•cin

sta•tus
s. anginosus

stax•is

steal
coronary s.
endoperoxide s.
subclavian s.

ste•a•rate

ste•a•ric acid

ste•ar•i•form

ste•a•rin

ste•a•ro•yl

ste•a•tog•e•nous

ste•a•tol•y•sis

ste•a•to•lyt•ic

ste•a•to•sis
  s. cardiaca

steel
  stainless s.

Steell
  Graham-S's murmur
  S's murmur

steg•no•sis

steg•not•ic

Stein•ert
  S's disease

stel•lec•to•my

steno•car•dia

steno•cho•ria

ste•no•sal

ste•nosed

ste•no•sis
  aortic s.
  aortic valve s.
  atherosclerotic aortic valvular s.
  bicuspid calcific aortic s.
  bifurcational s.
  buttonhole mitral s.
  calcific aortic s.
  calcific senile aortic s.
  calcified aortic s.
  caroticovertebral s.
  congenital aortic s.
  congenital dome aortic valve s.
  congenital mitral s.

ste•no•sis *(continued)*
  congenital valvular aortic s.
  coronary s.
  coronary artery s.
  diffuse calcific severe s.
  eccentric s.
  fibrous subaortic s.
  fishmouth mitral s.
  idiopathic hypertrophic subaortic s.
  infundibular s.
  left anterior descending artery s.
  membranous subvalvular aortic s.
  mitral s.
  muscular hypertrophic subaortic s.
  muscular subaortic s.
  myocardial infundibular s.
  peripheral pulmonic s.
  pulmonary s.
  pulmonary valve s.
  pulmonic s.
  pulmonic valvular s.
  rheumatic aortic s.
  silent mitral s.
  subaortic s.
  subpulmonic s.
  subvalvular s.
  subvalvular aortic s.
  supravalvular s.
  supravalvular aortic s.
  supraventricular aortic s.
  syphilitic coronary ostial s.
  tricuspid s.
  unicommissural aortic valve s.
  valvular s.
  valvular aortic s.
  vascular s.
  venous s.

ste•not•ic

step-down

stepped-care

step-up

Ster•a•pred

Stern
- S's position

ster•nal

ster•nal•gia

Stern•berg
- Albright-McCune-S. syndrome

ster•no•dyn•ia

ster•no•peri•car•di•al

ster•not•o•my
- median s.

ste•roid
- anabolic s.

ste•roid 11β-mono•oxy•gen•ase

ste•roid 17α-mono•oxy•gen•ase

ste•roid 21-mono•oxy•gen•ase

ste•rol

steth•acous•tic

steth•og•ra•phy

stetho•phone

stetho•pho•nom•e•ter

stetho•poly•scope

stetho•scope
- binaural s.
- Cammann's s.
- DeLee-Hillis obstetric s.
- differential s.
- electronic s.
- esophageal s.
- Leff s.
- nuclear s.

stetho•scop•ic

steth•os•co•py

Ste•vens
- Johnson-S. disease
- S.-Johnson syndrome

Ste•wart
- Hamilton-S. formula

STI
- systolic time intervals

stick
- sponge s.

Stick•ler
- S. syndrome

stiff•ness
- active dynamic s.
- cardiac s.
- cardiac muscle s.
- chamber s.
- chamber elastic s.
- diastolic s.
- elastic s.
- myocardial s.
- ventricular s.
- volume s.

stig•ma *pl.* stig•mas, stig•ma•ta
- peripheral s.

Still
- S's disease
- S's murmur

Stille
- S.-Giertz rib shears

Stil•phos•trol

stim•u•la•tion
- paired electrical s.
- programmed electrical s.
- vagal s.

stim•u•la•tor
- EP-2 Clinical S.

stim•u•lus *pl.* stim•u•li
- s. artifact
- atrial s.

stim•u•lus *(continued)*
depolarizing s.
electric s.
heterotopic s.
nomotopic s.
subthreshold s.
ventricular s.
ventricular electronic s.

sting
scorpion s.
scorpionfish s.
spider s.
wasp s.

ST in•ter•val

stitch
basting s.

stock•ings
compression s.
graded elastic compression s.
TED (thromboembolic disease) s.

Stokes
Adams-S. attack
Adams-S. syncope
Adams-S. syndrome
Cheyne-S. respiration
collar of S.
Morgagni-Adams-S. syndrome
S. syndrome
S.-Adams attack
S.-Adams syncope
S.-Adams syndrome

Sto•ma•to•coc•cus

stone
vein s.

stor•age
hypothermic s. for clinical heart preservation

storm
thyroid s.

Sto•vin
Hughes-S. syndrome

straight back syn•drome

strain

strand
drawn brazed s. (DBS)

Stratte
S. needle holder

Strauss
Churg-S. syndrome

streak
fatty s.

stream
axial s.

strength
tensile s.

strep•i•tus

Strep•tase

Strep•to•ba•cil•lus
S. moniliformis

Strep•to•coc•cus
S. pneumoniae

strep•to•coc•cus *pl.* strep•to•coc•ci

strep•to•ki•nase

strep•to•my•cin
s. sulfate

stress
left ventricular s.
left ventricular end-systolic s.
meridional wall s.
systolic wall s.
wall s.

stri•a•tion
tabby cat s.
tigroid s.

stric•ture
annular s.

stric•ture *(continued)*
contractile s.
recurrent s.

strip
rhythm s.

strip•per
Alexander rib s.
external vein s.
internal vein s.
Matson rib s.
rib s.
vein s.

stroke
back s.
embolic s.
heat s.

stron•ti•um
s.-82

strut
Elgiloy s.

ST seg•ment

study
biplane s.
Bogalusa Heart S.
cardiac electrophysiologic s.
Chicago People's Gas S.
Coronary Artery Surgery S. (CASS)
Doppler s.
ECG-gated s.
electrocardiogram-gated s.
electrophysiological s.
equilibrium s.
European Coronary Surgery S.
exercise thallium-201 s.
first pass s.
first pass dynamic radionuclide s.
first transit s.
Framingham Heart S.
gated blood pool s.

study *(continued)*
imaging s.
invasive electrophysiological s.
Los Angeles Heart S.
MUGA s.
multiple gated acquisition s.
myocardial perfusion s.
Oslo s.
planar stress-redistribution thallium-201 s.
Pooling Project S.
preoperative s.
radioisotopic s.
radionuclide s.
rest wall motion s.
resting thallium s.
resting wall motion s.
Seven Countries S.
single plane s.
stress thallium s.
stress wall motion s.
VA Cooperative S.
ventricular function s.
Veterans Administration Cooperative S.
wall motion s.
Western Electric S.
Zutphen S.

stun•ning
myocardial s.

Sturge
S.-Weber sequence

sty•let

sub•en•do•car•di•al

sub•epi•car•di•al

sub•in•ti•mal

Sub•li•maze

sub•scle•rot•ic

sub•stance
neurotransmitter s.

sub•stance *(continued)*
s. P

sub•thresh•old

sub•trac•tion
digital s.
functional s.
mask mode s.

sub•xi•phoid

suc•ci•nate

suc•ci•nyl•cho•line chlo•ride

Su•cos•trin

suc•tion
tonsil s.
Yankauer s.

su•fen•ta•nil

sul•cus *pl.* sul•ci
atrioventricular s.
s. coronarius cordis
coronary s. of heart
interventricular s., anterior
interventricular s., inferior
interventricular s., posterior
interventricular s. of heart
s. interventricularis anterior
s. interventricularis cordis
s. interventricularis inferior
s. interventricularis posterior
longitudinal s. of heart
longitudinal s. of heart, posterior
terminal s. of right atrium
s. terminalis atrii dextri
transverse s. of heart

sul•fa•di•a•zine

Sul•fa•meth•o•prim

sul•fa•meth•ox•a•zole

Sul•fa•prim

sul•fa•sal•a•zine

Sul•fa•trim

sul•fide
cupric s.
cuprous s.

sul•fin•py•ra•zone

sul•fi•sox•a•zole
s. acetyl
s. diolamine

sul•fo•lip•id

sul•fo•litho•cho•lyl•gly•cine

sul•fo•litho•cho•lyl•tau•rine

sul•fon•amide

sul•fo•nyl•urea

Sul•fox•a•prim

sul•fur
s. colloid
s. dioxide

sul•in•dac

sul•ma•zole

sum
ray s.

sump
left ventricular s.

su•per•fi•cial

su•pe•ri•or

su•per•i•or ve•na ca•val syn•drome

su•pero•lat•er•al

su•per•ox•ide

su•per•ox•ide dis•mu•tase

su•pine

sup•port
advanced cardiac life s.
advanced life s. (ALS)
advanced trauma life s.
basic life s. (BLS)
life s.

sup•pres•sion
overdrive s.

su•pra•cos•tal

su•pra•di•a•phrag•mat•ic

su•pra•val•var

su•pra•val•vu•lar

su•pra•ven•tric•u•lar

sur•face
anterior s. of heart
diaphragmatic s. of heart
endocardial s. of left ventricle
endocardial s. of right ventricle
inferior s. of heart
left s. of heart
right s. of heart
sternocostal s. of heart

sur•gery
ablative s.
aortocoronary bypass s.
bypass graft s.
cardiac s.
cardiothoracic s.
cardiovascular s.
compensatory s.
coronary artery s.
coronary artery bypass grafting s.
coronary bypass s.
excisional s.
noncardiac s.
open heart s.
reconstructive s.
reparative s.

Sur•gi•cel gauze

Sur•gi•lene suture

Sur•gi•lon suture

Sur•i•tal

Sur•mon•til

sur•vey
Jenkins Activity S.

sur•vi•val
long term s.
short term s.

Sus-Phrine

Sus•taire

su•sur•rus

su•ture
absorbable s.
absorbable surgical s.
atraumatic s.
braided s.
braided nylon s.
braided polyester s.
braided polyethylene fiber s.
braided silk s.
cannulation s.
cardiovascular s.
catgut s.
chromic catgut s.
chromic gut s.
collagen s.
continuous s.
cotton s.
Dacron s.
Dermalene s.
Dermalon s.
Dexon s.
double arm s.
Ethibond s.
Ethiflex s.
Ethilon s.
eyeless s.
fine s.
fine silk s.
Flexon s.
Flexon steel s.

su•ture *(continued)*
gut s.
gut s., chromic
gut s., plain
heavy silk s.
horizontal mattress s.
interrupted s.
s. ligature
linear polyethylene s.
mattress s.
Mersilene s.
monofilament s.
multifilament s.
Neurolon s.
nonabsorbable s.
nonabsorbable surgical s.
nylon s.
over-and-over s.
pericostal s's
Perma-Hand s.
plain gut s.
pledgeted s.
Polydek s.
polyester fiber s.
polyethylene s.
polyglactin 910 s.
polyglycolic acid s.
polypropylene s.
Prolene s.
pursestring s.
retention s.
retraction s.
running s.
silk s.
silk s., braided
silk s., fine
silk s., heavy
silk traction s.
stainless steel s.
stay s.
subcuticular s.
surgical steel s.
Surgilene s.
Surgilon s.
synthetic absorbable s.
Tevdek s.

su•ture *(continued)*
Ti-Cron s.
traction s.
uninterrupted s.
vertical mattress s.
Vicryl s.
wire s.

SVC
superior vena cava

$S\bar{v}O_2$
mixed venous oxygen saturation

SVR
systemic vascular resistance

SVT
supraventricular tachycardia

swaged

swal•low
Gastrografin s.

Swan
S.-Ganz catheter
S.-Ganz monitoring catheter

S wave

Sweet
S. sternal punch

switch
reed s.
voltage-sensitive s.

Sy•den•ham
S's chorea

Sylvius
valve of S.

sym•pa•thec•to•my
thoracic s.

sym•pa•thet•ic

sym•pa•tho•mi•met•ic

symp•tom
    Buerger's s.
    Oehler's s.
    prodromal s's

syn•chro•ny
    atrioventricular s.
    AV s.

syn•co•pe
    Adams-Stokes s.
    s. anginosa
    cardiac s.
    carotid sinus s.
    common s.
    deglutition s.
    electronic s.
    hysterical s.
    postmicturition s.
    post-tussive s.
    postural s.
    Stokes-Adams s.
    vasodepressor s.
    vasopressor s.
    vasovagal s.

syn•drome
    Aase s.
    acquired immunodeficiency s. (AIDS)
    Adams-Stokes s.
    adrenogenital s.
    adult respiratory distress s. (ARDS)
    AEC s.
    air entrapment s.
    Alagille's s.
    Albright's s.
    Albright-McCune-Sternberg s.
    Alport's s.
    ankyloblepharon-ectodermal dysplasia-clefting s.
    Antley-Bixler s.
    aortic arch s.
    aortic arteritis s.
    Apert's s.

syn•drome *(continued)*
    arteriohepatic dysplasia s.
    Ask-Upmark s.
    asplenia s.
    Babinski's s.
    Babinski-Vaquez s.
    Baller-Gerold s.
    ballooning mitral cusp s.
    Banti's s.
    Bardet-Biedl s.
    Barlow s.
    Bassen-Kornzweig s.
    Beals' s.
    Beals' contractural arachnodactyly s.
    Beau's s.
    Beckwith-Wiedemann s.
    Behçet's s.
    Bernheim's s.
    billowing mitral valve s.
    blepharophimosis s.
    blue toe s.
    Bouillaud's s.
    Bouveret's s.
    Brachmann-de Lange s.
    brachydactyly-spherophakia s.
    Bradbury-Eggleston s.
    bradycardia-tachycardia s.
    Canada-Cronkhite s.
    carcinoid s.
    cardiac-limb s.
    cardiofacial s.
    Carpenter's s.
    cat-eye s.
    Charcot's s.
    CHARGE association s.
    CHILD s.
    Chotzen's s.
    Churg-Strauss s.
    chylomicronemia s.
    click s.
    click murmur s.
    Cockayne's s.
    Coffin-Lowry s.
    Coffin-Siris s.
    Cohen's s.

syn•drome *(continued)*
- coloboma of iris–anal atresia s.
- concealed Wolff-Parkinson-White s.
- Conradi-Hünermann s.
- Cornelia de Lange's s.
- costosternal s.
- craniosynostosis–radial aplasia s.
- cri du chat s.
- Cronkhite-Canada s.
- cryptophthalmos s.
- Cushing's s.
- cutis laxa s.
- DaCosta's s.
- de Lange's s.
- DiGeorge s.
- Down s.
- Dressler's s.
- Ehlers-Danlos s.
- Eisenmenger's s.
- elfin facies s.
- Ellis-van Creveld s.
- euthyroid sick s.
- exomphalos-macroglossia-gigantism s.
- Fabry s.
- Fallot's s.
- familial deafness s.
- Fanconi's pancytopenia s.
- fetal alcohol s.
- fetal face s.
- fetal hydantoin s.
- fetal rubella s.
- fetal trimethadione s.
- fetal warfarin s.
- FG s.
- first and second branchial arch s.
- floppy valve s.
- Franceschetti-Klein s.
- Fraser s.
- Friedreich's s.
- G s.
- Gaisböck's s.
- Goldenhar's s.
- Goltz s.

syn•drome *(continued)*
- Gorlin's s.
- Gorlin-Goltz s.
- Gruber's s.
- Guillain-Barré s.
- Hamman-Rich s.
- Hay-Wells s.
- heart-hand s.
- Henoch-Schönlein s.
- holiday heart s.
- Holt-Oram s.
- homocystinuria s.
- Horton's s.
- Hughes-Stovin s.
- Hunter's s.
- Hunter-Hurler s.
- Hurler s.
- Hurler-Scheie compound s.
- Hutchinson-Gilford s.
- hypereosinophilic s.
- hyperkinetic heart s.
- hypersensitive carotid sinus s.
- hypertelorism-hypospadias s.
- hypomelia-hypotrichosis-facial hemangioma s.
- hypoplastic left-heart s.
- incontinentia pigmenti s.
- Ivemark's s.
- Jervell and Lange-Nielsen s.
- Kallmann's s.
- Kartagener's s.
- Kawasaki s.
- Kearns-Sayre s.
- Klein-Waardenburg s.
- Klippel-Feil s.
- LAMB (lentigenes, atrial myxoma, and blue nevi) s.
- Langer-Giedion s.
- Larsen's s.
- latent Wolff-Parkinson-White s.
- Laurence-Biedl s.
- Laurence-Moon-Biedl s.

syn•drome *(continued)*
Laurence-Moon-Biedl-Bardet s.
leopard s.
Leriche's s.
lethal multiple pterygium s.
Libman-Sacks s.
lissencephaly s.
Little's s.
long arm 18 deletion s.
long QT s.
low cardiac output s.
Lown-Ganong-Levine s.
Lutembacher's s.
McArdle s.
McCune-Albright s.
Mallory-Weiss s.
Marchesani's s.
Marfan s.
Maroteaux-Lamy s.
Maroteaux-Lamy mucopolysaccharidosis s.
Martorell's s.
Meckel's s.
Meckel-Gruber s.
midsystolic click s.
Minot-von Willebrand s.
mitral valve prolapse s.
Morgagni-Adams-Stokes s.
Morquio s.
Morquio-Ullrich s.
mucocutaneous lymph node s. (MLNS)
multiple lentigines s.
Nager s.
Nager acrofacial dysostosis s.
NAME (nevi, atrial myxoma, myxoid neurofibroma, ephelides) s.
Neu-Laxora s.
neurofibromatosis s.
non-Majewski type short rib–polydactyly s.

syn•drome *(continued)*
Noonan's s.
obesity-hypoventilation s.
old woman perforation s.
Opitz s.
Opitz-Frias s.
Ortner's s.
osteogenesis imperfecta s.
osteogenesis imperfecta s. type I
$4p^-$ s.
pacemaker s.
pacemaker twiddler's s.
painful pacemaker pocket s.
Pallister-Hall s.
pancytopenia-dysmelia s.
partial trisomy 10q s.
penta-X s.
Perheentupa s.
pericarditis-myocarditis s.
pickwickian s.
Polhemus-Schafer-Ivemark s.
polyangiitis overlap s.
polymyalgia rheumatica s.
polysplenia s.
postaxial acrofacial dysostosis s.
postcardiotomy psychosis s.
postcommissurotomy s.
post–myocardial infarction s.
postperfusion s.
postpericardiotomy s.
postphlebitic s.
postpump s.
post-thrombotic s.
preexcitation s.
progeria s.
prolapsed mitral valve s.
prolonged QT interval s.
pseudo-Hurler polydystrophy s.
pseudothalidomide s.
QT s.

syn•drome *(continued)*
radial aplasia–thrombocytopenia s.
red-neck s.
redundant cusp s.
Reiter's s.
Rendu-Osler-Weber s.
Riley-Day s.
Roberts-SC phocomelia s.
Robinow's s.
Romano-Ward s.
Rosenbach's s.
Roussy-Lévy s.
Rubinstein's s.
Rubinstein-Taybi s.
Ruvalcaba's s.
Saethre-Chotzen s.
scalenus anticus s.
Scheie's s.
Schinzel-Giedion s.
Schönlein-Henoch s.
scimitar s.
short PR s.
short rib–polydactyly s., non-Majewski type
Shprintzen's s.
Shy-Drager s.
sick sinus s.
sinoatrial s.
sinus s.
sleep apnea s.
sluggish sinus node s.
Sly s.
Smith-Lemli-Opitz s.
Spens' s.
spherophakia-brachymorphia s.
Stevens-Johnson s.
Stickler s.
"stiff heart" s.
straight back s.
subclavian steal s.
sudden infant death s.
superior vena cava s.
superior vena caval s.
supravalvular aortic stenosis s.
systolic click-murmur s.

syn•drome *(continued)*
Takayasu's s.
TAR s.
Taussig-Bing s.
thoracic outlet s.
thrombocytopenia–absent radius (TAR) s.
thromboembolic s.
Tietze's s.
Townes' s.
Treacher Collins s.
tridione s.
triploidy s.
trisomy 4p s.
trisomy 9 mosaic s.
trisomy 9p s.
trisomy 13 s.
trisomy 18 s.
trisomy 20p s.
trisomy 21 s.
Trousseau's s.
Turner's s.
Turner-like s.
twiddler's s.
Uhl's s.
Ullrich-Turner s.
vascular s.
vasculitis s.
velocardiofacial s.
von Willebrand's s.
Waardenburg's s.
Ward-Romano s.
Weber-Osler-Rendu s.
Weil's s.
Weill-Marchesani s.
Wellens' s.
Werner s.
Willebrand's s.
Williams s.
Wolff-Parkinson-White s.
WPW s.
XO s.
XXXX s.
XXXXX s.
XXXXY s.
XXXY s.
XXY s.

syn•drome *(continued)*
XYY s.

syn•ech•ia *pl.* syn•ech•iae
s. pericardii

syn•ge•ne•ic

syn•ge•ne•sio•plas•tic

syn•ge•ne•sio•trans•plan•ta•tion

syn•graft

Syn-Na•do•lol

Syn-Pin•do•lol

syn•vi•no•lin

syph•i•lis
cardiovascular s.

sy•ringe
disposable s.
glass s.
plastic s.
reusable s.
tuberculin s.

sys•tal•tic

sys•tem
adrenergic nervous s.
Advantz DX digital s.
automatic pacing s.
autonomic nervous s.
Bard Cardiopulmonary Support S.
blood-vascular s.
bulbospiral s.
cardiac conduction s.
cardiac pacing s.
cardiac parasympathetic nervous s.
cardinal venous s.
cardiovascular s.
central nervous s. (CNS)
central venous s.
chest drainage s.
circulatory s.
complement s.
conduction s. of heart

sys•tem *(continued)*
digital angiography s.
digital image review s.
excimer laser s.
fibrinolytic s.
fluid-filled catheter s.
Frank electrode s.
Frank lead s.
gated s.
hematopoietic s.
hexaxial reference s.
His-Purkinje s.
kallikrein-bradykinin s.
lead-electrode s.
metabolic equivalents s.
Mobin-Uddin filter s.
musculoskeletal s.
nervous s.
NTP s.
orthogonal lead s.
pacemaker code s.
pacing s.
parasympathetic nervous s.
phased-array echocardiography s.
Philips whole-body 4-Tesla magnetic resonance s.
plasma coagulation s.
portal s.
pressurized transducer s.
pulsatile pump s.
pump oxygenator s.
Purkinje s.
renin-angiotensin s.
renin-angiotension-aldosterone s.
reticuloendothelial s. (RES)
SDU-800 color cardiac ultrasound s.
SerialVue s.
Shaw monitoring s.
Siemens Coroskop C single plane angiocardiography s.
single plane angiocardiography s.

sys•tem *(continued)*
sinospiral s.
sympathetic nervous s.
sympathoadrenal s.
T s.
triaxial reference s.
underwater chest drainage s.
umbilicovitteline venous s.
Utah heart drive s.
Vario s.
vascular s.
vascular imaging s.
whole body angiography s.
Zoll NTP s.

sys•te•ma
s. conducens cordis

sys•to•le
aborted s.
atrial s.
electromechanical s.
extra s.
frustrate s.
total electromechanical s.
ventricular s.

sys•tol•ic

sys•to•lom•e•ter

T
  triggered (pacemaker code)

ta•ble
  fluoroscopic t.
  operating t.
  x-ray t.

TACE

tacho•gram

tach•og•ra•phy

tachy•ar•rhyth•mia
  supravalvular t.
  ventricular t.

tachy•car•dia
  antidromic t.
  antidromic circus movement t.
  atrial t.
  atrioventricular junctional reciprocating t.
  atrioventricular nodal t.
  atrioventricular nodal reentrant t.
  atrioventricular reciprocating t.
  automatic atrial t.
  benign ventricular t.
  bidirectional t.
  bidirectional ventricular t.
  bifascicular ventricular t.
  bundle branch reentrant t.
  chaotic atrial t.
  chronic nonparoxysmal sinus t.
  circus movement t.
  double t.
  ectopic t.
  fetal t.
  junctional t.

tachy•car•dia *(continued)*
  monomorphic ventricular t.
  multifocal atrial t.
  nodal t.
  nonparoxysmal t.
  nonparoxysmal atrioventricular junctional t.
  nonparoxysmal junctional t.
  nonsustained ventricular t.
  orthostatic t.
  pacemaker-mediated t.
  paroxysmal t.
  paroxysmal atrial t.
  paroxysmal junctional t.
  paroxysmal nodal t.
  paroxysmal reentrant supraventricular t.
  paroxysmal supraventricular t.
  paroxysmal ventricular t.
  polymorphic ventricular t.
  primary ventricular t.
  QRS t.
  reciprocating t.
  reentrant t.
  reflex t.
  refractory ischemic ventricular t.
  repetitive monomorphic ventricular t.
  sinoatrial nodal reeentrant t.
  sinus t.
  sinus nodal reentrant t.
  slow ventricular t.
  supranodal t.
  supraventricular t.
  sustained ventricular t.
  ventricular t.

tachy•car•dia *(continued)*
wide QRS t.

tachy•car•di•ac

tachy•car•dic

tachy•dys•rhyth•mia

tachy•pnea

tachy•rhyth•mia

tae•nia *pl.* tae•niae
t. terminalis

Tag•a•met

Ta•ka•ya•su
T's arteritis
T's disease
T's syndrome
T.-Ohnishi disease

talc

Tal•win

Tam•bo•cor

tam•bour

tam•pon•ade
cardiac t.
chronic t.
heart t.
low-pressure cardiac t.
pericardial t.

Tan•gier
T. disease

tan•ta•lum
t.-178

tape
cotton umbilical t.
lap t.
paper t.
silk t.
umbilical t.

Ta•per•cut needle

TAPVC
total anomalous pulmonary venous connection

TAR (radial aplasia–thrombocytopenia) syndrome

Ta seg•ment

tau•ro•che•no•de•oxy•cho•late

tau•ro•che•no•de•oxy•cho•lic acid

tau•ro•cho•late

tau•ro•cho•lic acid

Taus•sig
Blalock-T. anastomosis
Blalock-T. operation
Blalock-T. shunt
T.-Bing syndrome
T.-Bing type double-outlet right ventricle

Ta•wa•ra
node of Aschoff and T.
node of T.

Ta wave

Tay•bi
Rubinstein-T. syndrome

Tc
technetium

TE
echo delay time

Teb•ra•zid

Techne•Coll

Tech•ne•plex

Tech•ne•scan DTPA

Techne•Scan MAA

Techne•Scan PYP

tech•ne•ti•um
t. 99m

tech•ne•ti•um *(continued)*
t. Tc 99m albumin
t. Tc 99m albumin aggregated
t. Tc 99m carbomethoxy-isopropyl isonitrile
t. Tc 99m CPI
t. Tc 99m DTPA
t. Tc 99m glucoheptonate
t. Tc 99m isonitrile
t. Tc 99m methoxyisobutyl isonitrile
t. Tc 99m MIBI
t. Tc 99m pentetate
t. Tc 99m pertechnetate
t. Tc 99m (pyro- and trimeta-) phosphates
t. Tc 99m PYP
t. Tc 99m pyrophosphate
t. Tc 99m stannous pyrophosphate
t. Tc 99m sulfur colloid

Tech•ne•ti•um Tc 99m HSA

tech•ni•cian
pump t.

tech•nique
citrated bag blood harvesting t.
Creech t.
cryosurgical t.
digital subtraction t.
direct Fick t.
Dotter t.
dye dilution t.
fast low-angle shot t.
Fick t.
FLASH t.
GRASS (gradient-recalled acquisition in a steady state) t.
Gruentzig t.
heparinized blood harvesting t.
indicator dilution t.
indocyanine green indicator dilution t.

tech•nique *(continued)*
Judkins t.
kissing balloon t.
multipurpose catheter t.
Mustard t.
Rastelli t.
Seldinger t.
Sones t.
thermal dilution t.
thermodilution t.
Turbo FLASH (fast low-angle shot) t.
Vario t.

tech•nol•o•gist

TEDUS
transesophageal Doppler ultrasonography

TEE
transesophageal echocardiography

Tee•ba•co•nin

Tef•lon
T. catheter
T. cloth
T. felt
T. patch

TEG
thromboelastogram

Tega-Span

Teg•o•pen

Teg•re•tol

tel•an•gi•ec•ta•sia
hereditary hemorrhagic t.

tel•an•gi•ec•ta•sis *pl.* tel•an•gi•ec•ta•ses

tel•an•gi•ec•tat•ic

tel•an•gi•ec•to•des

tel•an•gi•on

tele•car•dio•gram

tele•car•di•og•ra•phy

tele•car•dio•phone

tele•di•ag•no•sis

tel•elec•tro•car•dio•gram

tel•elec•tro•car•dio•graph

tele•med•i•cine

tel•em•e•try
    cardiac t.

tel•es•theto•scope

Te•na•than

ten•do *pl.* ten•di•nes
    t. infundibuli

ten•don
    t. of conus
    coronary t's
    false t.
    t. of infundibulum
    t. of Todaro

Ten•ex

Ten•or•min

Ten•si•lon

ten•sion
    alveolar gas t.
    arterial t.
    arterial carbon dioxide t. ($PaCO_2$)
    arterial oxygen t. (PaO_2)
    intravenous t.
    left ventricular t.
    myocardial t.
    oxygen t.
    tissue t.
    wall t.

tep•ro•tide

te•ra•to•ma *pl.* te•ra•to•mas, te•ra•to•ma•ta
    cardiac t.

ter•bu•ta•line sul•fate

ter•mi•nal
    central t. of Wilson

ter•mi•na•tion
    underdrive t.

tes•la

test
    Allen's t.
    antistreptozyme t.
    Aschner's t.
    Aschner-Danini t.
    ASTZ t.
    atrial pacing stress t.
    Balke-Ware t.
    bicycle ergometer exercise t.
    blood coagulation t.
    capillary fragility t.
    capillary resistance t.
    cardiac MRI t.
    carotid sinus t.
    closed-ended t.
    cold pressor t.
    collateral circulation t.
    complement fixation t.
    Crampton's t.
    cuff t.
    cycle ergometer t.
    Dehio's t.
    dehydrocholate t.
    dexamethasone suppression t.
    ECG stress t.
    electrocardiographic stress t.
    ergometer exercise stress t.
    ergonovine t.
    exercise t's
    exercise thallium t.
    Gibbon and Landis t.
    graded exercise t.
    Göthlin's t.
    Hallion's t.
    Henle-Coenen t.
    Hess capillary t.
    Hines and Brown t.

test *(continued)*
hyperemia t.
indicator dilution t.
invasive t.
Korotkoff's t.
LAL t.
Lewis and Pickering t.
Liebermann-Burchard t.
limulus t.
limulus lysate t.
Limulus amoebocyte lysate t.
Machado t.
Machado-Guerreiro t.
Master step t.
Master "2-step" exercise t.
Master two-step exercise t.
Master two-step fitness t.
Matas' t.
maximal exercise t.
maximal treadmill t.
maximal treadmill stress t.
Mendelsohn's t.
modified Bruce t.
Moschcowitz t.
multistage bicycle ergometer t.
multistage treadmill t.
Naughton t.
noninvasive t.
noninvasive exercise stress t.
nuclide cardiac function t.
open-ended t.
Pachon's t.
Perthes' t.
plantar ischemia t.
pulmonary function t's
Quick tourniquet t.
Salkowski's t.
Sandrock t.
Schiff's t.
self-t.
Shultze's t.
standing plasma t.
stress t's

test *(continued)*
submaximal exercise t.
submaximal graded exercise t.
submaximal post–myocardial infarction t.
submaximal stress t.
thallium stress t.
tilt table t.
tolerance t.
tourniquet t.
treadmill t.
treadmill exercise t.
treadmill stress t.
Tuffier's t.
two-step t.
two-step exercise t.
ventilatory function t's
von Recklinghausen's t.
walking t.
whole blood coagulation time t. (WBCT)
Zwenger's t.

test•ing

tes•tos•te•rone

Te•su•loid

TET
treadmill exercise test

tet•ra•co•sa•no•ic acid

tet•ra•crot•ic

tet•ra•cy•cline
t. hydrochloride

tet•rad
Fallot's t.

te•tral•o•gy
t. of Eisenmenger
t. of Fallot

tet•ro•do•tox•in

Teut•le•ben
T's ligaments

Tev•dek
T. suture

TGV
transposition of the great vessels

thal•as•se•mia

tha•lid•o•mide

Tha•li•tone

thal•li•um
t.-201

THAM
tris(hydroxymethyl) aminomethane
tromethamine

the•be•si•an foramina

the•be•si•an valve

the•be•si•an veins

The•be•si•us
T. valve
veins of T.

the•ca *pl.* the•cae

Thee•lin

Theile
T's canal

Theo-24

Theo 250

Theo•bid

the•o•bro•mine

Theo•chron

Theo•clear

Theo•cot

Theo-Dur

Theo•lair

Theo•mar

The•on

the•oph•yl•line
t. ethylenediamine
t. olamine
t. sodium acetate
t. sodium glycinate

the•o•rem
Bayes' t.
Bernouilli's t.

the•o•ry
aging t. of atherosclerosis
Bayliss t.
closed circulation t.
closed-open circulation t.
encrustation t.
fast circulation t.
immunological t. of aging
metabolic t. of atherosclerosis
myogenic t.
open circulation t.
open-closed circulation t.
sliding filament t.

Theo•span

Theo-SR

Theo•stat

Theo-Time

Theo•vent

ther•a•py
antianginal t.
antiarrhythmic t.
antibiotic t.
antifibrinolytic t.
antihypertensive t.
antiplatelet t.
behavioral t.
combination t.
corticosteroid t.
diet t.
digitalis intoxication t.
diuretic t.
electrical ablation t.
fibrinolytic t.

ther•a•py *(continued)*
immunosuppressive t.
magnesium t.
medical t.
nondrug t.
oxygen t.
pacemaker t.
prostaglandin t.
protamine t.
radiation t.
thrombolytic t.
transcatheter t.
vasodilator t.

ther•mis•tor

ther•mo•di•lu•tion

ther•mo•pile
bismuth telluride t.

thi•a•mine

thi•am•y•lal so•di•um

thi•a•zide

thick•en•ing
cardiac wall t.
diffuse intimal t.
wall t.

thin•ning
apical t.

thio•cy•a•nate
t. sodium

Thio•mer•in

thio•na•mide

thio•pen•tal so•di•um

thio•rid•a•zine hy•dro•chlo•ride

Thom•sen
T's disease

tho•ra•cal

tho•rac•ic

tho•rac•ic out•let syn•drome

tho•ra•cot•o•my
left anterior t.

Tho•ra•dol

tho•rax *pl.* tho•ra•ces

Thor•a•zine

Tho•rel
T's bundle

Tho•ro•nil

Thor-Prom

THR
target heart rate

thresh•old
anaerobic t.
atrial pacing t.
capture t.
chronic ventricular t.
electrical stimulation t.
fibrillation t.
lactate t.
pacing t.
sensing t.
stimulation t.
stimulation energy t.
ventilatory t.
work t.

thrill
aneurysmal t.
aortic t.
diastolic t.
presystolic t.
purring t.
systolic t.

throm•bas•the•nia

throm•bec•to•my

throm•bem•bo•lia

throm•bi

throm•bin

throm•bo•an•gi•itis
t. obliterans

throm•bo•aor•top•a•thy
occlusive t.

throm•bo•ar•te•ri•tis
t. purulenta

throm•bo•ath•ero•scle•rot•ic

throm•boc•la•sis

throm•bo•clas•tic

throm•bo•cyst

throm•bo•cys•tis

throm•bo•cyte

throm•bo•cyt•ic

throm•bo•cy•to•pe•nia
essential t.

throm•bo•cy•to•poi•e•sis

throm•bo•cy•to•sis
primary t.

throm•bo•em•bo•lism
cerebral t.
pulmonary t.
venous t.

throm•bo•end•ar•ter•ec•to•my

throm•bo•end•ar•ter•itis

throm•bo•en•do•car•di•tis

throm•bo•gen•e•sis

throm•bo•gen•ic

β-throm•bo•glob•u•lin

throm•bo•ki•ne•sis

throm•bo•ki•net•ics

throm•bol•y•sis
coronary t.
intracoronary t.
intravenous t.

throm•bo•lyt•ic

throm•bo•mod•u•lin

throm•bo•pe•nia
essential t.

throm•bo•phil•ia

throm•bo•phle•bi•tis

throm•bo•plas•tic

throm•bo•plas•tid

throm•bo•plas•tin

throm•bo•poi•e•sis

throm•bo•poi•et•ic

throm•bosed

throm•bo•sis
acute coronary t.
agonal t.
aortic t.
arterial t.
cardiac t.
cerebral t.
coronary t.
creeping t.
deep vein t.
deep venous t. (DVT)
dilatation t.
left atrial appendage t.
mesenteric t.
plate t.
platelet t.
portal vein t.
propagating t.
recurrent occult systemic venous t.
Ribbert's t.
silent t.
traumatic t.
venous t.

throm•bos•ta•sis

throm•bot•ic

throm•box•ane
t. A2

throm•box•ane syn•thase

throm•box•ane syn•the•tase

throm•bus *pl.* throm•bi
  agonal t.
  agony t.
  annular t.
  antemortem t.
  atrial t.
  ball t.
  ball-valve t.
  blood plate t.
  blood platelet t.
  calcified t.
  cardiac t.
  coronary t.
  currant jelly t.
  endocardial t.
  hyaline t.
  intracardiac t.
  laminated t.
  lateral t.
  left atrial appendage t.
  left ventricular t.
  mixed t.
  mural t.
  obstructive t.
  occluding t.
  occlusive t.
  organized t.
  pale t.
  parietal t.
  postmortem t.
  primary t.
  propagated t.
  red t.
  stratified t.
  traumatic t.
  venous t.
  white t.

thump•ver•sion

thy•mo•ma

thy•ro•tox•i•co•sis
  neonatal t.

thy•rox•ine
  D-t.
  L-t.

Ti
  titanium

TIA
  transient ischemic attack

ti•ap•a•mil
  t. hydrochloride

Ti•car

ti•car•cil•lin
  t. cresyl sodium
  t. disodium

ti•clo•pi•dine hy•dro•chlo•ride

Ti-Cron su•ture

tie
  free t.
  heavy silk t.
  silk t.
  stick t.

Tiet•ze
  T's disease
  T's syndrome

tie-on-passer

TIG (tungsten–inert gas) weld•ing

tight•en•er
  wire t.

tim•bre
  t. métallique

time
  activated clotting t.
  aortic cross t.
  atrioventricular nodal conduction t.
  atrioventricular sequential t.
  circulation t.
  conduction t.
  dead t.
  echo delay t.
  His-Purkinje conduction t.

time *(continued)*
intra-atrial conduction t.
intra-atrioventricular nodal conduction t.
left ventricular ejection t.
lysis t.
magnetic relaxation t.
one-stage prothrombin t.
partial thromboplastin t. (PTT)
prothrombin t.
relaxation t.
repetition t.
R peak t.
sinoatrial conduction t.
sinus node recovery t.
thrombin t. (TT)
T2 relaxation t.

Ti•men•tin

tim•ing
escape interval t.

Ti•mo•lide

ti•mo•lol mal•e•ate

tin

tine
passive fixation t's

tip
Andrews suction t.
catheter t.
Frazier suction t.
glass t.
Luer-Lok needle t.
tonsil suction t.
Yankauer suction t.

Tip•ra•mine

tis•sue
adipose t.
atrioventricular junctional t.
automatic t.
AV junctional t.
conductile t.
conducting t.

tis•sue *(continued)*
connective t.
contractile t.
fatty t.
junctional t.
nodal t.
subcutaneous t.

tis•sue plas•min•o•gen ac•ti•va•tor

ti•ta•ni•um
t. disulfide

ti•tra•tor

Tl
thallium

TMST
treadmill stress test

TNF
tumor necrosis factor

to•bra•my•cin
t. sulfate

to•cai•nide
t. hydrochloride

to•coph•er•ol
α-t.
alpha-t.

To•daro
tendon of T.

TOF
tetralogy of Fallot

To•fra•nil

tol•az•o•line hy•dro•chlo•ride

tol•er•ance
acquired immune t.
exercise t.
immune t.

to•mog•ra•phy
automatic computerized axial t.
cine computed t.
computed t.

to•mog•ra•phy *(continued)*
computerized axial t. (CAT)
emission t.
high-resolution computerized t.
gated computed t.
positron emission t. (PET)
rapid-acquisition computer-assisted t.
single-photon emission computed t. (SPECT)
technetium pyrophosphate single-photon emission computed t.
thallium-201 t.
ultrasonic t.

tone
heart t's
Traube's double t.

Tono•card

to•nog•ra•phy
carotid compression t.

to•nom•e•ter
Gärtner's t.
Recklinghausen's t.

To•nom•i•tor

ton•sil•lo•ad•e•noid•ec•to•my

Tooth
Charcot-Marie-T. disease

tor•sades de pointes

Tor•u•lop•sis
T. glabrata

to•rus *pl.* to•ri
t. aorticus

To•ta•cil•lin

tour•ni•quet
automatic rotating t.
Esmarch's t.

tour•ni•quet *(continued)*
pneumatic t.
Rumel t.

Townes
T. syndrome

tox•emia

tox•in

tox•o•plas•mo•sis

TPA
tissue plasminogen activator

tPA
tissue plasminogen activator

t-PA
tissue plasminogen activator
tissue-type plasminogen activator

T-Phyl

TPR
temperature, pulse, and respiration

T-Quil

TR
repetition time

tra•bec•u•la *pl.* tra•bec•u•lae
trabeculae carneae cordis
trabeculae cordis
fleshy trabeculae of heart
septomarginal t.
t. septomarginalis

tra•bec•u•lo•plas•ty

trac•er
positron-emitting t.
radioactive t.

trac•ing
carotid pulse t.
jugular venous pressure t.

trac•ing *(continued)*
jugular venous pulse t.
M-mode t.
pressure t.
venous pulse t.

tract
atrio-His t.
atriohisian t's
atrioventricular bypass t's
flow t.
flow t. of the heart
inflow t.
internodal t's
left ventricular outflow t.
outflow t.
right ventricular outflow t.
Wolff-Parkinson-White bypass t.

Tran•date

tran•qui•liz•er

trans•an•nu•lar

trans•aor•tic

trans•atri•al

trans•cap•il•lary

Trans•derm-Nitro

Trans•derm-Scōp

Trans•derm-V

trans•du•cer
diaphragm t.
echo t.
pressure t.

tran•sect

tran•sec•tion

trans•esoph•a•ge•al

trans•fer•rin

trans•for•ma•tion
Fourier t.

trans•fu•sion
blood t.

trans•lu•mi•nal

trans•me•dia•sti•nal

trans•me•di•as•ti•nos•co•py

trans•mi•tral

trans•mu•ral

trans•plant
cardiac t.
heart t.
heart-lung t.
lung t.
pulmonary t.

trans•plan•ta•tion
allogeneic t.
bone marrow t.
cardiac t.
heart t.
heart-lung t.
heterologous t.
heterotopic t.
homologous t.
organ t.
orthotopic t.
syngenesioplastic t.

trans•port
monovalent cation t.
reverse cholesterol t.

trans•po•si•tion
congenitally corrected t. of great vessels
D-t. of the great arteries
t. of great arteries
t. of great vessels
L-t. of the great arteries
partial t. of great vessels

trans•sep•tal

trans•tele•phon•ic

trans•tho•rac•ic

trans•ve•nous

trans•ven•tric•u•lar

tran•yl•cy•pro•mine sul•fate

Tra•si•cor

Tras•y•lol

Traube
T's double tone
T's heart
T's membrane
T's murmur
T's sign
T's space
T.-Hering waves

trau•ma *pl.* trau•mas, trau•ma•ta
blunt t.

tra•zo•done hy•dro•chlo•ride

Tra•zon

Trea•cher Col•lins
T.C. syndrome
T.C.-Franceschetti syndrome

tread•mill
Naughton cardiac exercise t.

treat•ment
Fränkel's t.

trem•or
t. cordis
purring t.

Tren•del•en•burg
T's operation
T's test

trend•scrib•er

trend•scrip•tion

Tren•tal

trep•i•da•tio
t. cordis

tre•pop•nea

trep•pe

tri•ac•yl•glyc•er•ol

tri•ac•yl•glyc•er•ol li•pase

tri•ad
acute compression t.
Beck's t.
Kartagener's t.
Osler's t.

Tri•ad•a•pin

tri•al
Australian Therapeutic T.
Coronary Primary Prevention T. (CPPT)
Lipid Research Clinics Coronary Primary Prevention T.
Medical Research Council T.
MILIS t.
MRC T.
Multicenter Investigation for the Limitation of Infarct Size t.
Multiple Risk Factor Intervention T. (MRFIT)

Tria•lo•dine

tri•am•ter•ene

tri•an•gle
t. of auscultation
Burger's scalene t.
cardiohepatic t.
Einthoven's t.
femoral t.
Gerhardt's t.
t. of Koch
t. of safety

tri•a•zo•lam

Tri•az•ole

Tri-B3

trich•i•no•sis

Tri•chlor•ex

tri•chlor•me•thi•a•zide

tricho•car•dia

Tri•chos•po•ron

tri•crot•ic

tri•cro•tism

tri•cus•pid

Tri•dil

tri•di•one syn•drome

tri•fi•lar

tri•gem•i•ny

tri•glyc•er•ide

Tri•glyc•er•ide Con•sen•sus Con•fer•ence

tri•gone
fibrous t. of heart, left
fibrous t. of heart, right

tri•go•num *pl.* tri•go•na
t. fibrosum dextrum cordis
t. fibrosum sinistrum cordis

tri•io•do•thy•ro•nine

Trik•acide

tril•o•gy
t. of Fallot

tri•ma•zo•sin hy•dro•chlo•ride

tri•met•a•phan
t. camsylate

tri•meth•o•prim
t. sulfate

Tri•meth-Sul•fa

tri•mip•ra•mine
t. maleate

Tri•mox

Trim•pex

tri•o•le•in

tri•pal•mi•tin

tri•phen•yl•tet•ra•zo•li•um
t. chloride

tri•ploi•dy syn•drome

tri•pod
Haller's t.

Trip•til

tri•pus
t. halleri

tris(hy•droxy•meth•yl)•am•i•no•meth•ane

tri•so•my
t. 4p
t. 9 mosaic
t. 9p
t. 13
t. 18
t. 20p
t. 21

tri•stea•rin

Tri•sul•fam

tro•car
t. needle

Tro•lard
T's net
T's plexus

tro•meth•amine

tro•po•my•o•sin

tro•po•nin
t. C
t. I
t. T

trou•sers
military (medical) anti-shock t. (MAST)

Trous•seau
T's syndrome

trun•cus *pl.* trun•ci
t. arteriosus

trun•cus *(continued)*
t. arteriosus, persistent
t. brachiocephalicus
t. coeliacus
t. costocervicalis
t. externa vasorum
t. externa vasorum [adventitia]
t. fasciculi atrioventricularis
partial t. arteriosus
persistent t. arteriosus
t. pulmonalis
t. thyreocervicalis
t. thyrocervicalis

trunk
t. of atrioventricular bundle
t. of bundle of His
celiac t.
pulmonary t.

Tru•phyl•line

Trux•o•phyl•lin

Try•pan•o•so•ma
T. cruzi
T. rhodesiense

try•pano•so•mi•a•sis
acute t.
African t.
chronic t.

TSC

TTC (triphenyltetrazolium chloride) stain•ing

TTI
tension-time index

Tu•ba•rine

Tubbs
T. mitral valve dilator

tube
bifurcated t.
cathode-ray t.
chest t.

tube *(continued)*
double-lumen t.
Mallinckrodt right-sided double-lumen t.
straight t.

tu•ber•cle
intervenous t.
intravascular t.
Lower's t.

tu•ber•cu•lo•sis
renal t.

tu•ber•cu•lum *pl.* tu•ber•cu•la
t. intervenosum
t. intervenosum [Loweri]
t. Loweri

tub•ing
pump t.
rubber t.
vinyl t.

tu•bo•cu•ra•rine
t. chloride

tu•bule
convoluted t's
distal convoluted t.
proximal t.
proximal convoluted t.

Tuf•fier
T's test

tug•ging
tracheal t.

tu•men•tia
vasomotor t.

tu•mor
atrial t.
carcinoid t.
cardiac t.
cardiac granular cell t.
cardiac thyroid t.
papillary t.
varicose t.

tung•sten

tu•nic
    Bichat's t.

tu•ni•ca *pl.* tu•ni•cae
    t. adventitia vasorum
    t. elastica interna
    t. intima vasorum
    t. media vasorum

tun•nel
    aortico-left ventricular t.

Turbo FLASH (fast low-angle shot) technique

tur•bu•lence

Tur•ner
    T's syndrome
    Ullrich-T. syndrome

Tur•ner-like syndrome

T wave

twid•dler's syn•drome

twist•er
    wire t.

type
    Duchenne's t.

ty•phus
    scrub t.

typ•ing
    HLA t.

ty•ra•mine

U

U
  uranium

Ud•din
  Mobin-U. filter
  Mobin-U. filter system

Uhl
  U's anomaly
  U's syndrome

ul•cer
  atheromatous u.
  hypertensive ischemic u.
  peptic u.
  stasis u.
  varicose u.

Ull•rich
  Morquio-U. syndrome
  U.-Turner syndrome

ul•ti•mum mo•ri•ens

Ul•tra•cef

ul•tra•cen•trif•u•ga•tion

ul•tra•fil•tra•tion

ul•tra•sono•gram

ul•tra•sono•graph•ic

ul•tra•so•nog•ra•phy
  A-mode u.
  B-mode u.
  continuous wave Doppler u.
  CW (continuous wave) Doppler u.
  Doppler u.
  pulsed u.
  pulsed reflected u.
  pulsed wave Doppler u.
  PW (pulsed wave) Doppler u.

ul•tra•sono•scope

ul•tra•sound
  Doppler u.
  three-dimensional u.

un•der•sens•ing

un•du•la•tion
  jugular u.

uni•fo•cal

Uni•gen

Uni•pen

Uni•phyl

uni•po•lar

unit
  coronary care u.
  digital fluoroscopic u.
  general care u.
  intensive care u.
  Life Change U's
  Life Support U.
  peripheral resistance u. (PRU)
  resistance u.
  Wood u.

Up•mark
  Ask-U. syndrome

up•stroke
  diastolic u.

up•take
  lung thallium-201 u.
  oxygen u.

Ura•beth

ura•ni•um

ura•pi•dil

urea
  blood u. nitrogen (BUN)

Ure•cho•line

ure•mia

ure·thane
polyether u.

ur·gen·cy
hypertensive u.

uric acid

Uri·don

uri·nal·y·sis

Uri·tol

Uro·cit-K

uro·ki·nase

Uro·plus

Uro·vist

Uro·zide

ur·so·de·oxy·cho·late

ur·so·de·oxy·cho·lic acid

ur·so·de·oxy·cho·lyl·gly·cine

ur·so·de·oxy·cho·lyl·tau·rine

US Army retractor

USP
United States Pharmacopeia

USP gauge

Utah
U. artificial heart
U. heart drive system
U. pneumatic heart driver

U wave

V

V
  vanadium

V
  voltage

VA
  Veterans Administration

vac•cen•ic acid

vac•cine
  streptococcal v.
  streptococcus v.

vac•cin•ia

VA Co•op•er•a•tive Study

va•gi•na *pl.* va•gi•nae
  v. vasorum

va•go•lyt•ic

va•go•mi•met•ic

va•go•ton•ic

V–A in•ter•val

Val•er•gen

Val•i•um

Val•re•lease

Val•sal•va
  V's experiment
  V's maneuver
  sinus of V.

val•ue
  resting v.

val•va *pl.* val•vae
  v. aortae
  v. aortica
  v. atrioventricularis dextra
  v. atrioventricularis sinistra
  v. mitralis

val•va *(continued)*
  v. pulmonaria
  v. tricuspidalis
  v. trunci pulmonalis

val•val

val•var

val•vate

valve
  v. of aorta
  aortic v.
  artificial v.
  artificial cardiac v.
  atrioventricular v., left
  atrioventricular v., right
  auriculoventricular v., left
  auriculoventricular v., right
  backbleed v.
  ball v.
  Beall prosthetic v.
  Beall-Surgitool prosthetic v.
  bicuspid v.
  bicuspid aortic v.
  bioprosthetic v.
  Björk-Shiley v.
  Björk-Shiley convexoconcave prosthetic v.
  Björk-Shiley monostrut prosthetic v.
  Björk-Shiley prosthetic v.
  Braunwald-Cutter prosthetic v.
  BS (Björk-Shiley) prosthetic v.
  caged-ball v.
  cardiac v's
  cardiac v., artificial
  Carpentier-Edwards v.
  caval v.

valve *(continued)*
convexoconcave prosthetic v.
Cooley-Cutter caged-disk v.
coronary v.
v. of coronary sinus
Cross-Jones prosthetic v.
DeBakey-Surgitool prosthetic v.
double-orifice mitral v.
Duromedics bileaflet v.
eccentric monocusp v.
eustachian v.
flail mitral v.
flail tricuspid v.
flair v.
v. of foramen ovale
Hall-Kaster prosthetic v.
Hancock v.
Hancock bioprosthetic v.
Hancock porcine prosthetic v.
Harken prosthetic v.
heart v's
heart v., artificial
v. of inferior vena cava
interauricular v.
Ionescu v.
Ionescu-Shiley pericardial v.
Ionescu-Shiley prosthetic v.
Kay-Shiley prosthetic v.
Kay-Suzuki prosthetic v.
Lillehei-Kaster pivoting-disk v.
Lillehei-Kaster prosthetic v.
Magovern-Cromie prosthetic v.
Meadox-Gabbay unicusp pericardial v.
mechanical v.
Medtronic-Hall v.
Medtronic-Hall prosthetic v.

valve *(continued)*
Medtronic-Hall tilting-disk v.
MH (Medtronic-Hall) prosthetic v.
mitral v.
monostrut v.
Omnicarbon tilting-disk v.
Omniscience tilting-disk v.
parachute mitral v.
pivoting-disk v.
porcine v.
porcine heterograft v.
porcine prosthetic v.
prosthetic v.
pulmonary v.
pulmonary trunk v.
v. of pulmonary trunk
pyrolytic carbon disk v.
rheumatic tricuspid v.
St. Jude Medical bileaflet v.
SE (Starr-Edwards) prosthetic v.
semilunar v.
SJ (St. Jude Medical) prosthetic v.
Smeloff-Cutter prosthetic v.
Starr-Edwards v.
Starr-Edwards caged-ball v.
Starr-Edwards prosthetic v.
stenotic v.
Surgitool prosthetic v.
v. of Sylvius
thebesian v.
tilting-disk v.
tissue v.
tricuspid v.
trileaflet aortic v.
v. of veins
Wada-Cutter prosthetic v.

valved

val•vi•form

val•vo•tome

val•vot•o•my
Brock v.
closed v.
mitral v.
pulmonary v.
transventricular closed v.

val•vu•la *pl.* val•vu•lae
v. foraminis ovalis
v. mitralis
v. semilunaris
v. semilunaris anterior trunci pulmonalis
v. semilunaris dextra aortae
v. semilunaris dextra trunci pulmonalis
v. semilunaris posterior aortae
v. semilunaris sinistra aortae
v. semilunaris sinistra trunci pulmonalis
v. sinus coronarii
v. sinus coronarii [Thebesii]
v. venae cavae inferioris
v. venae cavae inferioris [Eustachii]
v. venosa

val•vu•lar

val•vule

val•vu•li•tis
aortic v.
mitral v.
rheumatic v.
syphilitic aortic v.

val•vu•lo•plas•ty
aortic v.
balloon v.
intracoronary thrombolysis balloon v.
mitral v.
percutaneous balloon v.

val•vu•lo•plas•ty *(continued)*
percutaneous transluminal balloon v.
pulmonary v.

val•vu•lo•tome

val•vu•lot•o•my
pulmonary v.

va•na•di•um

Van•co•cin

Van•co•led

van•co•my•cin hy•dro•chlo•ride

Van•cor

van Cre•veld
Ellis-v.C. syndrome

Vapo-Iso

Va•quez
Babinski-V. syndrome

var•i•a•tion
paradoxical respiratory v.

var•i•ca•tion

var•i•ce•al

var•i•cel•la

var•i•ces

var•ic•i•form

var•i•coid

var•i•cose

var•i•co•sis

var•i•cos•i•ty

var•i•cot•o•my

Va•rio
V. program
V. system
V. technique
V. voltage threshold–measuring pulse generator

va•ri•o•la

var•ix *pl.* var•i•ces
anastomotic v.
aneurysmal v.
aneurysmoid v.
arterial v.
cirsoid v.

vas *pl.* va•sa
vasa brevia
v. capillare
vasa intestini tenuis
vasa nervorum
vasa nutritia
v. sinusoideum
vasa vasorum

va•sal

va•sal•gia

vas•cu•lar

vas•cu•lar•i•ty

vas•cu•lar•iza•tion

vas•cu•lar•ize

vas•cu•la•ture

vas•cu•lit•ic

vas•cu•li•tis
allergic v.
hypersensitivity v.
leukocytoclastic v.
livedo v.
necrotizing v.
nodular v.
overlap v.
pulmonary v.
segmented hyalinizing v.

vas•cu•lo•gen•ic

vas•cu•lo•lym•phat•ic

vas•cu•lo•mo•tor

vas•cu•lop•a•thy

vas•cu•lo•tox•ic

vas•cu•lum *pl.* vas•cu•la

va•sec•to•my

Vas•er•et•ic

vas•i•fac•tive

vas•i•form

vaso•ac•tive

vaso•con•stric•tion
pulmonary v.

vaso•con•stric•tive

vaso•con•stric•tor

vaso•co•ro•na

vaso•de•pres•sion

vaso•de•pres•sor

vaso•di•la•ta•tion

vaso•di•la•tion
reflex v.

vaso•di•la•tive

vaso•di•la•tor
balanced v.

vaso•fac•tive

vaso•for•ma•tive

vaso•gan•gli•on

vaso•hy•per•ton•ic

vaso•hy•po•ton•ic

vaso•in•ert

vaso•mo•tion

vaso•mo•tor

vaso•mo•to•ri•al

vaso•mo•tor•ic•i•ty

vaso•mo•to•ri•um

vaso•mo•to•ry

vaso•neu•rop•a•thy

vaso•neu•ro•sis

vaso•pa•re•sis

vaso•per•me•a•bil•i•ty

vaso•pres•sin
  arginine v. (AVP)

vaso•pres•sor

vaso•re•lax•a•tion

vaso•spasm
  coronary artery v.

vaso•spas•mo•lyt•ic

vaso•spas•tic

vaso•stim•u•lant

Vaso•tec

vaso•to•nia

vaso•ton•ic

vaso•tribe

vaso•trip•sy

vaso•troph•ic

Vas•ox•yl

VAT (atrial synchronous ventricular) pace•maker

VAT (atrial synchronous ventricular) pac•ing

VATER (vertebral defects, imperforate anus, transesophageal fistula, and radial and renal dysplasia) as•so•ci•a•tion

Va•ze•pam

VB
  ventricular bradycardia

VCG
  vectorcardiogram
  vectorcardiography

VDD (atrial-synchronous ventricular-paced) pace•maker

VDD (atrial-synchronous ventricular-paced) pac•ing

vec•tor
  P v.
  QRS v.
  T v.

vec•tor•car•dio•gram

vec•tor•car•dio•graph

vec•tor•car•di•og•ra•phy
  spatial v.

vec•tor•scope

ve•cu•ro•ni•um

veg•e•ta•tion
  bacterial v's
  verrucous v's

vein
  accompanying v.
  adrenal v's
  afferent v's
  anonymous v's
  antebrachial v., median
  appendicular v.
  arterial v.
  arterial v. of Soemmering
  atrial v's of heart
  atrioventricular v's of heart
  axillary v.
  azygos v.
  azygos v., left
  azygos v., lesser superior
  basilic v.
  basilic v., median
  basivertebral v's
  brachial v's
  brachiocephalic v's
  bronchial v's
  Burow's v.
  cardiac v's
  cardiac v's, anterior
  cardiac v., great
  cardiac v., middle
  cardiac v., small
  cardiac v's, smallest
  central v.

vein *(continued)*
central v's of hepatic lobules
central v's of liver
central v. of suprarenal gland
cephalic v.
cephalic v., accessory
cephalic v., median
cervical v., deep
cervical v's, transverse
circumflex femoral v's, lateral
circumflex femoral v's, medial
circumflex iliac v., deep
circumflex iliac v., superficial
colic v., left
colic v., middle
colic v., right
common cardinal v's
common femoral v.
communicating v's
coronary v., left
costoaxillary v's
cubital v., median
cutaneous v., ulnar
cystic v.
deep v.
deep v. of thigh
dorsispinal v's
epigastric v., inferior
epigastric v., superficial
epigastric v's, superior
epiploic v., left
epiploic v., right
esophageal v's
femoral v.
femoral v., deep
femoropopliteal v.
fibular v's
gastric v., left
gastric v., right
gastric v's, short
gastroepiploic v., left
gastroepiploic v., right
gastro-omental v., left

vein *(continued)*
gastro-omental v., right
genicular v's
gluteal v's, inferior
gluteal v's, superior
hemiazygos v.
hemiazygos v., accessory
hepatic v's
hepatic v's, intermediate
hepatic v's, left
hepatic v's, middle
hepatic v's, right
hypogastric v.
hypophyseoportal v's
ileal v's
ileocolic v.
iliac v., common
iliac v., external
iliac v., internal
iliolumbar v.
v's of inferior member, deep
v's of inferior member, superficial
infralobar v.
infrasegmental v.
innominate v's
intercostal v's, anterior
intercostal v., highest
intercostal v's, posterior
intercostal v., superior, left
intercostal v., superior, right
interlobar v's of kidney
interlobular v's of kidney
interlobular v's of liver
intermediate v.
intersegmental v.
intervertebral v.
jejunal v's
jugular v., anterior
jugular v., anterior horizontal
jugular v., external
jugular v., internal
v's of kidney
Krukenberg's v's

vein *(continued)*
laryngeal v., inferior
laryngeal v., superior
v's of lower member, deep
v's of lower member, superficial
lumbar v's
lumbar v., ascending
mammary v's, external
mammary v., internal
v. of Marshall
Marshall's oblique v.
median v. of elbow
median v. of forearm
median v. of neck
mediastinal v's
mesenteric v., inferior
mesenteric v., superior
musculophrenic v's
oblique v. of left atrium
obturator v's
oesophageal v's
ovarian v., left
ovarian v., right
pancreatic v's
pancreaticoduodenal v's
paraumbilical v's
parumbilical v's
perforating v's
pericardiac v's
pericardiacophrenic v's
peroneal v's
phrenic v's, inferior
phrenic v's, superior
popliteal v.
portal v.
portal v. of liver
posterior v. of left ventricle
prepyloric v.
pudendal v's, external
pudendal v., internal
pulmonary v's
pulmonary v., left inferior
pulmonary v., right inferior
pulmonary v., left superior

vein *(continued)*
pulmonary v., right superior
pyloric v.
radial v's
radial v., external, of Soemmering
renal v's
Retzius's v's
sacral v's, lateral
sacral v., middle
saphenous v.
saphenous v., accessory
saphenous v., great
saphenous v., small
v's of Sappey
small v. of heart
spinal v's, anterior and posterior
splenic v.
sternocleidomastoid v.
v. stripper
subclavian v.
subcostal v.
sublobular v's
submental v.
superficial v.
superficial femoral v.
v's of superior member, deep
v's of superior member, superficial
suprarenal v., left
suprarenal v., right
suprascapular v.
thebesian v's
v's of Thebesius
thoracic v's, internal
thoracic v., lateral
thoracoacromial v.
thoracoepigastric v's
thyroid v., inferior
thyroid v's, middle
thyroid v., superior
tibial v's, anterior
tibial v's, posterior
transverse v's of neck
ulnar v's

vein *(continued)*
- umbilical v.
- v's of upper member, deep
- v's of upper member, superficial
- uterine v's
- ventricular v's of heart
- vertebral v.
- vertebral v., accessory
- vertebral v., anterior
- vertebral v's, superficial
- v's of vertebral column
- v's of vertebral column, external
- v's of Vieussens

ve•lo•car•dio•fa•cial syn•drome

ve•lo•cim•e•try
- laser-Doppler v.

ve•loc•i•ty
- conduction v.
- mean v. of circumferential fiber shortening

Vel•o•sef

ve•na *pl.* ve•nae
- venae anonymae [dextra et sinistra]
- v. appendicularis
- venae atriales cordis
- venae atrioventriculares cordis
- v. axillaris
- v. azygos
- v. basilica
- venae basivertebrales
- venae brachiales
- venae brachiocephalicae (dextra/sinistra)
- venae bronchiales
- venae bronchiales anteriores
- venae bronchiales posteriores
- venae cardiacae anteriores
- v. cardiaca magna

ve•na *(continued)*
- v. cardiaca media
- venae cardiacae minimae
- v. cardiaca parva
- v. cava
- venae cavae
- v. cava inferior
- v. cava superior
- v. cava superior, persistent left
- v. centralis glandulae suprarenalis
- venae centrales hepatis
- v. cephalica
- v. cephalica accessoria
- v. cervicalis profunda
- venae circumflexae femoris laterales
- venae circumflexae femoris mediales
- v. circumflexa iliaca profunda
- v. circumflexa ilium profunda
- v. circumflexa ilium superficialis
- venae circumflexae laterales femoris
- venae circumflexae mediales femoris
- v. circumflexa superficialis ilium
- v. colica dextra
- v. colica intermedia
- v. colica media
- v. colica sinistra
- venae columnae vertebralis
- v. comitans
- venae comitantes arteriae femoralis
- venae cordis
- venae cordis anteriores
- v. cordis magna
- v. cordis media
- venae cordis minimae
- v. cordis parva
- venae costoaxillares

ve•na *(continued)*
v. cystica
v. epigastrica inferior
v. epigastrica superficialis
venae epigastricae superiores
v. epiploica dextra
v. epiploica sinistra
venae esophageae
venae esophageales
v. femoralis
v. femoropoplitea
venae fibulares
venae gastricae breves
v. gastrica dextra
v. gastrica sinistra
v. gastroepiploica dextra
v. gastroepiploica sinistra
v. gastro-omentalis dextra
v. gastro-omentalis sinistra
venae geniculares
venae genus
venae gluteae inferiores
venae gluteae superiores
v. hemiazygos
v. hemiazygos accessoria
venae hepaticae
venae hepaticae dextrae
venae hepaticae intermediae
venae hepaticae mediae
venae hepaticae sinistrae
v. hypogastrica
venae ileales
v. ileocolica
v. iliaca communis
v. iliaca externa
v. iliaca interna
v. iliolumbalis
inferior v. cava
venae intercostales
venae intercostales anteriores
venae intercostales posteriores
v. intercostalis superior dextra

ve•na *(continued)*
v. intercostalis superior sinistra
v. intercostalis suprema
venae interlobares renis
venae interlobulares hepatis
venae interlobulares renis
v. intermedia antebrachii
v. intermedia basilica
v. intermedia cephalica
v. intermedia cubiti
vena intervertebralis
venae jejunales
v. jugularis anterior
v. jugularis externa
v. jugularis interna
v. laryngea inferior
v. laryngea superior
v. lienalis
venae lumbales
v. lumbalis ascendens
v. mammaria interna
v. mediana antebrachii
v. mediana basilica
v. mediana cephalica
v. mediana colli
v. mediana cubiti
venae mediastinales
venae mediastinales anteriores
v. mesenterica inferior
v. mesenterica superior
venae musculophrenicae
v. obliqua atrii sinistri
v. obliqua atrii sinistri [Marshalli]
venae obturatoriae
venae oesophageales
v. ovarica dextra
v. ovarica sinistra
venae pancreaticae
venae pancreaticoduodenales
venae paraumbilicales
venae parumbilicales [Sappeyi]
venae pectorales

ve•na *(continued)*
venae perforantes
venae pericardiacae
venae pericardiacophrenicae
venae pericardiales
venae peroneae
venae phrenicae inferiores
venae phrenicae superiores
v. poplitea
v. portae hepatis
v. portalis hepatis
v. posterior ventriculi sinistri cordis
v. prepylorica
vena profunda
v. profunda femoris
venae profundae membri inferioris
venae profundae membri superioris
venae pudendae externae
v. pudenda interna
venae pulmonales
v. pulmonalis dextra inferior
v. pulmonalis dextra superior
v. pulmonalis inferior dextra
v. pulmonalis inferior sinistra
v. pulmonalis sinistra inferior
v. pulmonalis sinistra superior
v. pulmonalis superior dextra
v. pulmonalis superior sinistra
venae radiales
venae renales
venae renis
venae sacrales laterales
v. sacralis media
v. sacralis mediana
v. saphena accessoria

ve•na *(continued)*
v. saphena magna
v. saphena parva
v. scapularis dorsalis
venae spinales anteriores/posteriores
v. splenica
v. sternocleidomastoidea
v. subclavia
v. subcostalis
v. superficialis
venae superficiales membri inferioris
venae superficiales membri superioris
superior v. cava
v. suprarenalis dextra
v. suprarenalis sinistra
v. suprascapularis
v. thoracalis lateralis
venae thoracicae internae
v. thoracica lateralis
v. thoracoacromialis
venae thoracoepigastricae
v. thyreoidea ima
venae thyreoideae inferiores
venae thyreoideae superiores
v. thyroidea inferior
venae thyroideae mediae
v. thyroidea superior
venae tibiales anteriores
venae tibiales posteriores
venae transversae cervicis
venae transversae colli
v. transversa scapulae
venae ulnares
v. umbilicalis
venae uterinae
venae ventriculares cordis
v. vertebralis
v. vertebralis accessoria
v. vertebralis anterior

ve•na•ca•vo•gram

ve•na•ca•vog•ra•phy

ve•nae

ve•na•tion

ve•nec•ta•sia

ve•nec•to•my

vene•punc•ture

vene•sec•tion

vene•su•ture

veni•punc•ture

veni•sec•tion

veni•su•ture

ve•no•atri•al

ve•no•au•ric•u•lar

ve•no•con•stric•tion

ve•no•fi•bro•sis

ve•no•gram

ve•nog•ra•phy

ve•no•mo•tor

ve•no-oc•clu•sive

ve•no•pres•sor

ve•no•scle•ro•sis

ve•nose

ve•no•si•nal

ve•nos•i•ty

ve•no•sta•sis

ve•not•o•my

ve•nous

ve•no•ve•nos•to•my

vent
Sarns v.

ven•ti•la•tion
arterial v.
mechanical v.

ven•ti•la•tor
positive-pressure v.

Ven•to•lin

ven•trad

ven•tral

ven•tri•cle
aortic v. of heart
atrialized right v.
auxiliary v.
congenital single v.
double-outlet v.
double-outlet left v.
double-outlet right v.
v. of heart
left v. of heart
right v. of heart
single v.
Taussig-Bing type double-outlet right v.

ven•tric•u•lar

ven•tric•u•lar•i•za•tion

ven•tric•u•lo•gram

ven•tric•u•log•ra•phy
blood pool radionuclide v.
contrast v.
direct v.
equilibrium radionuclide v.
exercise radionuclide v.
first pass v.
gated blood pool v.
gated radionuclide v.
intravenous v.
isotope v.
left v.
radioisotope v.
radionuclide v.
radionuclide stress v.

ven•tric•u•lo•my•ot•o•my

ven•tric•u•lo•nec•tor

ven•tric•u•lot•o•my
encircling endocardial v.

ven•tric•u•lot•o•my *(continued)*
partial encircling endocardial v.

ven•tric•u•lus *pl.* ven•tric•u•li
v. cordis
v. dexter cordis
v. sinister cordis

ven•trim•e•son

ven•tro•dor•sad

ven•tro•dor•sal

ven•tro•lat•er•al

ven•tro•me•di•an

ven•tro•pos•te•ri•or

Ven•turi
V. effect

ven•tu•rim•e•ter

ven•u•la *pl.* ven•u•lae

ven•u•lar

ven•ule

ven•u•li•tis

Ve•Pe•sid

ver•ap•a•mil
v. hydrochloride

Ver•e•lan

Ver•neuil
V's canal

ver•te•bro•ar•te•ri•al

ver•te•bro•bas•i•lar

ver•tex *pl.* ver•ti•ces
v. cordis

ve•sic•u•lo•tu•bu•lar

ve•sic•u•lo•tym•pan•ic

ves•sel
aortopulmonary collateral v.

ves•sel *(continued)*
arterioluminal v's
arteriosinusoidal v's
blood v.
collateral v.
coronary collateral v.
ghost v.
great v's
nutrient v's
sinusoidal v.

ves•ti•bule
v. of aorta
Sibson's v.

Vet•er•ans Ad•min•is•tra•tion Co•op•er•a•tive Study

VFib
ventricular fibrillation

Vfib
ventricular fibrillation

VFL
ventricular flutter

VFl
ventricular flutter

V-Gan

VHDL
very-high-density lipoprotein

vi•a•bil•i•ty
myocardial v.

vi•bro•car•dio•gram

vi•bro•car•di•og•ra•phy

vi•bro•pho•no•car•dio•graph

Vi•cryl su•ture

vi•deo•den•si•to•met•ric

vi•deo•den•si•tom•e•try

Vie•us•sens
V. annulus
V. ansa
V. foramina
isthmus of V.

Vie•us•sens *(continued)*
limbus of V.
ring of V.
veins of V.

vil•lus *pl.* vil•li
pericardial v.

Vin•ca•sar

Vin•crex

vin•cris•tine sul•fate

Vine•berg
V. operation

vi•rus
Coxsackie A v.
Coxsackie B v.
ECHO v.
Epstein-Barr v. (EB v., EBV)
human immunodeficiency v. (HIV)
respiratory syncytial v.
vaccinia v.

vis•co•sim•e•ter
Ostwald v.

vis•cos•i•ty
blood v.

Vis•ken

Vi•ta•graft arteriovenous shunt

vi•ta•min
v. B
v. B_1
v. D
v. K

Vi•ta•tron impulse analyzer

vit•i•li•go
symmetric v.

vit•i•um *pl.* vit•ia
v. cordis

Vi•vac•til

Vi•vol

VLDL
very-low-density lipoprotein

β-VLDL
β-very-low-density lipoprotein

Volk•mann
V's ischemic paralysis
V. retractor

vol•ume
blood v.
cardiac v.
circulating v.
circulation v.
v. of circulation
v. of distribution
end-diastolic v.
end-expiratory lung v.
end-systolic v.
forward stroke v.
intravascular v.
left ventricular v.
left ventricular end-diastolic v.
left ventricular stroke v.
mean corpuscular v.
right ventricular v.
stroke v.

vom•it•ing

von Reck•ling•hau•sen
v.R's disease
v.R's test

von Wil•le•brand
Minot-v.W. syndrome
v.W.'s blood coagulation factor
v.W.'s disease
v.W.'s syndrome

VOO (ventricular asynchronous) pace•maker

VOO (ventricular asynchronous) pac•ing

voo•doo death

vor•tex *pl.* vor•ti•ces
- v. cordis
- v. of heart

VPB
- ventricular premature beat

VPC
- ventricular premature contraction
- ventricular premature complex

VSD
- ventricular septal defect

VT
- ventricular tachycardia

V TACH
- ventricular tachycardia

VTach
- ventricular tachycardia

VVI (ventricular demand inhibited) pace•maker

VVI (ventricular inhibited) pac•ing

VVIR (ventricular demand inhibited–rate responsive) pace•maker

VVI-RR (ventricular demand inhibited–rate responsive) pace•maker

VVT (ventricular demand triggered) pace•maker

VVT (ventricular triggered) pac•ing

v wave

vWf
- von Willebrand's factor

W

W
tungsten

Waar•den•burg
Klein-W. syndrome
W's syndrome

Wäch•ter
Bracht-W. bodies
Bracht-W. lesion

Wag•en•er
Keith-W.-Barker classification

wall
free w.

Wan•gi•el•la

WAP
wandering atrial pacemaker

Ward
Romano-W. syndrome
W.-Romano syndrome

Ware
Balke-W. protocol
Balke-W. test

war•fa•rin
w. sodium

War•fi•lone

wash•out
lactate w.
thallium w.

wast•ing
potassium w.
salt w.

Wa•ta•na•be
W. heritable hyperlipidemic (WHHL) rabbit

Wa•ter•ston
W. operation

Wa•ter•ston *(continued)*
W. shunt

watt

watt-se•cond

wave
A w.
a w.
afterpotential w.
anacrotic w.
anadicrotic w.
c w.
cannon a w's
capacitor discharge w.
catacrotic w.
catadicrotic w.
cove-plane T w.
cv w.
delta w's
depolarizing w.
dicrotic w.
F w's
f w's
fibrillary w's
flutter w's
giant a w's
H w.
h w.
J w.
Mayer w's
non-Q w.
notched, bifid T w.
Osborne w.
P w.
papillary w.
percussion w.
pressure w.
pulse w.
Q w.
R w.
rapid filling w.
recoil w.
regurgitant w's
S w.

wave *(continued)*
- sine w.
- skipped P w.
- slow filling w.
- T w.
- Ta w.
- tidal w.
- Traube-Hering w's
- tricrotic w.
- U w.
- v w.
- ventricular w.
- x w.
- y w.

wave•form
- pressure w.

WBCT
- whole blood coagulation time

Web•er
- Osler-W.-Rendu disease
- Sturge-W. sequence
- W.-Osler-Rendu syndrome

Wed•en•sky
- W. inhibition

wedge
- passive fixation w.

We•ge•ner
- W's granulomatosis

Weh•gen

Weil
- W's disease
- W's syndrome

Weill
- W.-Marchesani syndrome

Wein•berg
- W. retractor

Weiss
- Haber-W. reaction
- Mallory-W. syndrome

Weit•lan•er
- W. retractor

Well•bu•trin

Wel•lens
- W. syndrome

Wells
- Hay-W. syndrome

Wen•cke•bach
- W. block
- W. cycle
- W. exit block
- W. heart block
- W. period
- W. phenomenon
- W. second degree heart block

Werl•hof
- W's disease

Wer•ner
- W's syndrome

West•berg
- W's space

Wes•tern Elec•tric Study

Wh
- watt-hour

WHHL (Watanabe heritable hyperlipidemic) rab•bit

Whip•ple
- W's disease

White
- McGinn-W. sign
- Wolff-Parkinson-W. bypass tract
- Wolff-Parkinson-W. (WPW) syndrome

WHO
- World Health Organization

width
- pulse w.

Wiede•mann
- Beckwith-W. syndrome

Wig•gers
  W. diagram

Wil•le•brand
  Minot-W. syndrome
  W's blood coagulation factor
  W's disease
  W's syndrome

Wil•liams
  W. syndrome

Wil•son
  central terminal of W.
  W's leads

win•dow
  aortic w.
  aorticopulmonary w.
  aortic-pulmonary w.
  aortopulmonary w.
  biological w.
  cycle-length w.
  subxiphoid pericardial w.

Win•i•war•ter
  W.-Buerger disease

Win•pred

Wint•ro•cin

wire
  exchange w.
  lead w.

Wolff
  concealed W.-Parkinson-White syndrome
  latent W.-Parkinson-White syndrome
  W. integrating pneumotachograph
  W.-Parkinson-White bypass tract
  W.-Parkinson-White (WPW) syndrome

Wol•vek
  W. sternal approximation fixation instrument

Wood
  Crile-W. needle holder
  W. unit

work
  stroke w.
  threshold w.

WPW (Wolff-Parkinson-White) syndrome

Wris•berg
  W's ganglion

Wya•my•cin

Wy•cil•lin

Wy•mox

Wy•ten•sin

Xan•ax

xan•thel•as•ma

xan•thine

xan•tho•ma
 eruptive x.
 palmar x.
 planar x.
 x. striatum palmare
 x. tendinosum
 tendinous x.
 tendon x.
 tuberoeruptive x.
 tuberous x.
 tuboeruptive x.

xan•tho•ma•to•sis
 cerebrotendinous x.

Xe
 xenon

xeno•di•ag•no•sis

xeno•graft
 cardiac x.

xeno•graft *(continued)*
 Hancock porcine x.

xe•non
 x. Xe 127
 x. Xe 133

xeno•trans•plan•ta•tion
 cardiac x.

XO syndrome

x-ray

x wave

XXXX syn•drome

XXXXX syn•drome

XXXXY syn•drome

XXXY syn•drome

XXY syn•drome

Xy•lo•caine

XYY syn•drome

XYZ leads

Y

Y
    yttrium

Yan·kau·er
    Y. suction
    Y. suction tip

year
    patient-y.

yeast

Yer·sin·ia

yt·tri·um

y wave

Z

Zahn
    pockets of Z.

Za•pex

Za•rox•o•lyn

Zec•nil

Zes•to•ret•ic

Zes•tril

Zet•ran

zinc

Zn
    zinc

Zol•i•cef

Zoll NTP system

zo•na *pl.* zo•nae
    zonae tendinosae cordis

zone
    infarct z.
    ischemic risk z.
    risk z.
    subendocardial z.
    tendinous z's of heart
    transitional cell z.

Zuck•er•kan•dl
    Z's bodies
    Z's gland
    organs of Z.

Zut•phen Study